The
Open-Focus®
B R A I N

The
Open-Focus®
BRAIN

Harnessing the Power of
Attention to Heal Mind and Body

Les Fehmi, PhD, and Jim Robbins

TRUMPETER
BOSTON & LONDON / 2008

This book is not intended to substitute for medical advice or treatment.

TRUMPETER BOOKS
An imprint of Shambhala Publications, Inc.
Horticultural Hall
300 Massachusetts Avenue
Boston, Massachusetts 02115
www.shambhala.com

9 8 7 6 5 4 3

Printed in the United States of America

♾ This edition is printed on acid-free paper that meets
the American National Standards Institute z39.48 Standard.
♻ This book was printed on 30% postconsumer recycled paper.
For more information please visit www.shambhala.com.
Distributed in the United States by Random House, Inc.,
and in Canada by Random House of Canada Ltd

Designed by DCDESIGN

Library of Congress Cataloging-in-Publication Data

Fehmi, Les.
The open-focus brain: harnessing the power of attention
to heal mind and body / Les Fehmi and Jim Robbins.
        p.   cm.
Includes bibliographical references and index.
ISBN 978-1-59030-376-4 (hardcover: alk. paper)
ISBN 978-1-59030-612-3 (paperback: alk. paper)
1. Psychology—Miscellanea. 2. Attention—
Physiological aspects. I. Robbins, Jim. II. Title.
RC480.5.O6443 2007
616.89—dc22
2006103033

Compared to what we ought to be, we are only half awake. Our fires are damped, our drafts are checked. We are making use of only a small part of our possible mental and physical resources.

— WILLIAM JAMES, from an address to the American Philosophical Association, Columbia University, 1906

Contents

Contents

Preface

THE HUMAN mind is essential to life as we know it. Everything created by humans—from artwork to architecture to automobiles to our school systems and foreign policy—has its origin in the mind. Critical decisions—whether to go to war, what to create, whether to protect the environment, what to buy and sell—virtually everything—are based on decisions made by a human mind. The health and well-being of our civilization, it could be argued, rests on the health and well-being of our central nervous system and its offspring, the mind.

But the mind is a funny thing. We assume, if we think about it, that our mind is what it is, and there's little we can do—or should do—to change it. And because we may have lived with anxiety or depression or ADD for so long, we may not realize how serious our problem is or what life is like without it.

But we have all had expansive experiences. We may have traveled to Europe or backpacked in Yellowstone or stayed for a week at summer camp or fallen in love, or have done all of those things. And when we come back from these expansive experiences we feel different.

These experiences are more than fleeting bouts of pleasure or momentary lapses in the anxiety or depression or boredom of the stressful lives we endure the rest of the time. They show that we can move out of the flat, two-dimensional world that is all too often our daily life into a broad, multidimensional range of sensations, perceptions, and awareness that we only experience once in a while.

The question, of course, is how to make these changes. There are a number of different approaches, from religious faith to yoga to meditation to medications to exercise to the arts.

Another is neurofeedback, a very simple computerized form of biofeedback that allows the user to gain control of his or her brain waves simply by being able to see on a computer screen what their brain waves are doing. I was stunned by how well something as simple as neurofeedback could treat attention-deficit/hyperactivity disorder (ADHD), anxiety, depression, and a host of other ailments and wrote about it in my 2000 book, *A Symphony in the Brain: The Evolution of the New Brain-Wave Biofeedback*.

In 1998, while researching that book, I walked into Les Fehmi and Susan Shor Fehmi's office, a warren of rooms full of wires and strobe lights and CD players, and had Les place five saline sensors of his neurofeedback equipment on my head.

The concept is simple. Fehmi's brain-wave biofeedback—which he calls brain-wave synchrony training—is little more than a sophisticated mirror that lets your brain see what it's doing when you are producing specific brain waves that are the hallmark of specific forms of attention that Fehmi calls "Open Focus."

For half an hour I sat in a chair with my eyes closed, receiving light and sound feedback. I also listened to a tape of what Fehmi calls guided "imageless imagery." It didn't take conscious effort—the central nervous system responds automatically to this special form of light-and-sound feedback. Fifteen minutes into the very first session I could feel changes taking place. Clenched muscles that I didn't know were clenched were letting go, and a calm settled over me. When I stood up I was slightly disoriented and knew a great deal of stress had been released. I wanted more. Fehmi gave me several recorded Open-Focus exercises and told me to listen to them twice a day. "But three times a day," he said, "is like a bottle rocket."

Like many people, I had become habituated to the stress I carried. I didn't know how bad it was until I began to release it.

Open-Focus attention changed many things for me and for the people whose stories are presented in this book. It was during an exercise with Fehmi that I finally understood the essence of Open Focus. As I sat in a chair, Fehmi showed me a reproduction of *Christina's World*, the well-known painting by Andrew Wyeth. It depicts a girl reclining in a field who looks toward a house in the distance. As I looked at the painting, I saw Christina as foreground and everything else—the grass field she was crawling across, the house and shed and sky—as background. After a twenty-minute, eyes-closed Open-Focus exercise, I relaxed and looked at the painting again: It was a revelation. This time my eyes took in the whole painting simultaneously: Christina, the field, the house, and the sky were all one whole picture. My eyes didn't go from her to the house to the shed to the sky. It was a subtle but dramatic difference. I knew then that I wanted to write a book about attention and how it shapes awareness.

Many journalists get into the business because they want to right the wrongs they see in the world. That was certainly my motivation. I started reporting on the environment. And I wrote about severely abused children. As a journalist I've always striven to get above ground level to look at the big picture, and so to discern the root causes of our problems.

In the last ten years or so I have come to realize that many— if not most—of the grievous problems we face spring, in large part, from the same source. We are a species and a culture that, through our attention habits, carry past wounds that cause anger, fear, longing, and sorrow. These affect our lives far more deeply than we realize. We see the world through an imperfect lens, which deeply colors our perceptions, making us more angry, fearful, sorrowful, and overwhelmed than we need to be. Our attention habits, and the emotions they repress, keep us separate from the world, from feeling part of it; they prevent us from fully sensing what is around us and participating in it. As a result, we are unable to fully engage the here and now. The cruel irony is that because we have no other frame of reference, because we do not pay attention to how we pay attention, we think we are seeing the world as it is.

But we have the power to change. It starts with how we pay attention. Les Fehmi has made an important discovery about the role of attention in human behavior and physiology, and it should open a new dialogue about the human condition.

— JIM ROBBINS

Acknowledgments

M y DEEPEST gratitude to Susan Shor Fehmi, whose sustained personal support, clinical expertise, and literary contributions to this work were immeasurably important to me. She is credited with the material provided in the chapter on attention and psychotherapy.

Many thanks to Professors Ron Johnson and Jim McGaugh for rescuing me from a comparatively dry career in physics and math.

Many thanks also to Professor Donald B. Lindsley at the UCLA Brain Research Institute for opening his laboratories to me and providing the first inkling that the physiological correlates of attention were important.

My gratitude to Joshu Sasaki Roshi, who inspired me to make the subject of awareness and attention my personal quest as well, and for keeping my will, interest, and effort alive by not accepting my answers to his koans.

My gratitude to my children, Laura, Jeffrey, and Emy Fehmi, for many critical comments and positive suggestions.

My gratitude to Phyllis Loften for years of administrative assistance in completing this work. Thanks also to Lawrence Kettlekamp for his contributions to an earlier manuscript.

Many thanks to our copy editor, Jacob Morris, for his knowledgeable and thoughtful editing; to our assistant editor,

Acknowledgments

Ben Gleason, for many valued suggestions; and to our insight-ful editor, Eden Steinberg, who acquired the book and made a significant contribution to its shape and scope; and to our agent, Stuart Bernstein, who brought the manuscript to Eden's attention and who mentored us all the way to publication.

— Les Fehmi

The
Open-Focus®
B R A I N

Introduction

*There is more to life than
increasing its speed.*

— MOHANDAS K. GANDHI

I F Y O U are like most people these days, Gandhi's warning has probably gone unheeded and the speed of life seems to be increasing exponentially. Many clients tell me they rush through the day—dropping the kids off at school, zipping off to work on jam-packed freeways, frantically playing out in their heads the things they need to do, obsessing over the details of work or school, juggling cell-phone calls as they drive—anxious to cram as much as they can into their lives lest they miss something.

But many people also tell me that even when they stop rushing about, they can't wind down. They complain of not being able to fall asleep or of feeling edgy, irritable, anxious, depressed, restless, impatient, dissatisfied, or bored—or all of the above. They can't relax unless they have a drink or two. During the day they have trouble mustering the energy to focus and pay attention, and so they power up with double espressos. They have headaches, backaches, and a long list of other chronic physical problems. Thoughts race through their heads. And many people say they feel they are merely skimming the surface of what goes on around them, missing out on the deeper feelings of life's experiences.

These kinds of problems are epidemic. But in most cases there is nothing wrong with the people who suffer them; nor is anything necessarily wrong with their lives. Instead it is a matter of "operator error." Everyone has the ability to rebalance and heal their nervous systems to end these problems, to dissolve their pain, to slow down and yet accomplish more, to experience life more deeply, to optimize the function of their bodies and minds, to dramatically change their lives for the better. They just don't know how.

The answer is simple and well within their grasp—it is accomplished by changing the way they pay attention.

When I ask someone how they pay attention, they usually scratch their head and wonder what I mean. Most people assume they are paying attention or not, end of story. There exists little vocabulary to describe, and scant physiology to understand, how we pay attention. At first glance the subject, quite honestly, seems dull.

For more than forty years, however, I have been a student of how human beings attend both to the world around them and to their internal world of emotions and thoughts. Pry beneath the surface of the subject of attention, and there is a fascinating and fundamental phenomenon that has intrigued holy men, psychologists, military researchers, and advertising executives for many years. And for good reason: attention is the central mechanism through which we guide our awareness and experience the world.

The term "paying attention" is an apt one, for too often it is more costly than we realize. Failing to deploy our attention appropriately can cost us dearly by contributing to a host of physiological and emotional problems and keeping us from reaching our full potential. The truth is that most of us go through life paying attention the wrong way.

For the past thirty years people have come to our workshops and to our clinic, the Princeton Biofeedback Center, in Princeton, New Jersey, to learn one thing: how to change the way they pay attention. Without drugs or other medical interventions, people from all walks of life learn to reduce stress; dissolve chronic pain; stop anxiety; alleviate depression; ease fears, shame, envy, anger, and loneliness; and overcome attention deficit disorder (ADD), attention-deficit/hyperactivity disorder (ADHD), and other cognitive problems. The world-class executives, athletes, artists, and performers I've worked with have learned to dramatically improve their performance. And other health professionals have come to learn to apply the lessons of attention to everything from psychotherapy to massage.

The changes that come from learning to pay attention in different ways aren't subtle—they have robust effects on the entire nervous system, from our eyes to our muscles to our mind, body, and spirit. Here are some examples:

- Mary had a twenty-year history of chronic physical problems, the worst of which were severe migraine headaches that occurred almost daily and sometimes lasted for three days. After several months of Open-Focus training, Mary reported that the headaches had been reduced to fewer than one per month. She was able to take a new job and took up long-distance running. "I feel like the world is my place again," she says happily.
- For most of his adult life Aaron suffered ulcerative colitis, a condition that causes extreme pain in the large intestine, accompanied by fatigue and loss of appetite. He was in

3

constant discomfort, seldom traveled, and could only eat certain foods. After Open-Focus training his illness vanished completely, and he started traveling and eating in restaurants again.

- Thomas was a trumpet player who suffered extreme performance anxiety before his auditions for Broadway musicals and in jazz clubs. It was taking a toll on his ability to make a living and ruined the enjoyment he got from playing. Through attention training he learned to let go, relax, and yet be centered in the creative presentation of his talent. His playing became more spontaneous and smooth. "I found I could be more present in the moment, which is what good music is all about," he said.

- Tristan, a New Jersey mother, was so gripped by panic attacks and agoraphobia (fear of public spaces) that she was unable to leave her home. These attacks came on suddenly and out of nowhere, causing her heart to race, stealing her breath, and making her feel faint. She started Open-Focus training, and her fears and panic attacks diminished and were eventually eliminated.

My interest in the power of attention began during a research fellowship in 1969 at the NASA Ames Research Center at Moffett Field, California, when I developed a kidney stone. One afternoon a sudden, shuddering pain, unlike anything I had ever felt, rippled through my body and almost dropped me to the floor. Pain medications didn't help. Distracting myself didn't help; nor did creating a competing pain—bending back my finger or pinching myself. The pain bored through everything. Several hours later it disappeared as suddenly as it had arrived.

When the pain returned a few days later, I tried a new tack and did something that seemed counterintuitive: I searched out the precise location of the core of pain in my body and gave it my full attention. Then, instead of fighting it, which I had been doing consciously and unconsciously, I surrendered to it. I allowed myself not only to fully feel it but also to bathe in it and completely dive into and accept it. Immediately the pain ceased, and a wonderful feeling of lightness took its place. The world around me grew brighter, and I felt more present and centered. To my astonishment the pain was gone for a full day.

The next day, when the kidney-stone pain returned, the brightness dimmed. Again I stopped fighting it and dove into the pain. And again the same bright, clear feeling appeared. I formed my first hypothesis about what was going on: A major factor in how much pain I experienced was related to how I paid attention to it. Instead of focusing intently on the pain and fighting it, or focusing away and distracting myself, the trick was to pay attention in a way that put the pain squarely at the center of attention while I remained relaxed and broadly immersed in it with other senses present in the periphery of attention. Then the pain became a small part of my total awareness, rather than most or all of it, which allowed me to immerse this awareness—which is me—in the pain and let it diffuse and dissolve.

I was astonished that even pain this physical, this searing, could be brought under control—without medication, without surgery—simply by changing the way I paid attention to it. This discovery began a lifelong quest to understand the relationship between how people attend to the world and the profound effect that different forms of attention have on our minds and bodies. Decades later I have learned one overriding lesson: When we change the way we pay attention, we gain the power to profoundly change the way we relate to our world on every level—physically, emotionally, mentally, and spiritually.

The power of attention is no secret to the world of Eastern

spiritual disciplines and martial arts; they understood long ago that bringing attention under conscious control is a powerful way of mastering our internal and external realities. But our culture does not appreciate the role of attention in healing everything from depression to anxiety to ADD and ADHD, to myriad kinds of chronic pain and distress, sleep problems, fatigue, sadness, isolation, and irritability. We don't understand the role of attention in allowing us to experience true union. The most critical element of human experience is relationship, ranging from deep, loving connections with other people to feelings of oneness and union with the world. Learning to bring our attention under conscious control is how we optimize those relationships.

In 1998, Jim Robbins, a science journalist, walked into our office in Manhattan to interview me and my wife and partner, Susan Shor Fehmi, and to try Open-Focus techniques. Brainwave biofeedback, or neurofeedback—which feeds back signals to the user about the electrical activity of the brain and allows them to guide their brains into beneficial patterns of electrical activity—has been around as an effective treatment for anxiety and other problems since the 1960s. Computers enhanced its effectiveness in the 1980s, and today many different kinds of biofeedback and neurofeedback are used by thousands of practitioners around the world though it is not as well known as it should be because it falls outside the traditional medical model of care (medications and surgery).

Robbins also interviewed me because I was active in the early days of biofeedback. I chaired the first symposium of biofeedback researchers in 1968, and I helped found the Biofeedback Society of America in 1969, which later became the Association for Applied Physiology and Biofeedback. The AAPB now has more than two thousand members worldwide, and I continue to teach workshops at their annual meetings and at other professional meetings.

Open Focus is important because virtually everyone can learn to improve their attention skills and in turn their physiology. Learning to master our central nervous systems and with it our personal reality, through the use of optional attention skills, is the ultimate control and freedom.

There are many self-help books on the shelf these days. I find most of them to be vague and ineffective and lacking in specifics. That is one thing that I hope sets this book apart. As a clinician who has treated thousands of clients with neuro-feedback and Open-Focus attention training, I have spent decades perfecting specific exercises that can help people optimize their attention and get the most out of life.

The present book examines the crucial and global role that attention plays in our mind and body and explains, in concise language, the source of the healing and stress-reducing power of attention. Being aware of and using a variety of attention styles offers some of the same benefits offered by meditation but is based on scientific observation and research and is described in simple, everyday behavioral and physiological language. This book presents numerous exercises that allow readers to embark on a healing journey. If Open-Focus exercises become a routine practice, most readers will be able to learn to quickly dissolve all kinds of chronic emotional and physical pain and the discomfort of unwanted experience.

The Open-Focus Brain is first and foremost an optimistic book. The physicist Werner Heisenberg once said that what scientists observe "is not nature itself, but nature exposed to our method of questioning." When it comes to trying to understand the brain, researchers start with a strongly biased question: "What is *wrong* with the brain?" We need to abandon the biased view of the human central nervous system as somehow genetically and chemically flawed and the belief that a growing number of powerful drugs, whose mechanisms and long-term effects remain disturbingly unknown, will fix us. Instead we need to ask what is *right* with the nervous system and how we can enhance it by reducing operator errors. The best treatment tool for many, in my view, is attention training. The misuse and rigidity of attention get most of us into the chronic problems of anxiety, depression, and pain, and the effective use of attention skills can get us out. Flexible attention may not fix everything, but it can do far more than most imagine.

Humans were never meant to see the world through a lens of chronic fear or other negative emotions. We were meant to experience the world directly as it really is. We were meant to form deep connections to other human beings. With attention training at work, school, or home, we can open our hearts, experience the fullness of our senses, and reconnect with forgotten parts of ourselves. We can experience moments of unity and transcendence and find the world has been reenchanted. It will be a watershed moment in human evolution when we are able to pay attention to how we pay attention, control our attention, and take personal responsibility for the creation of our own realities. This is a truly profound realization, a revelation. It's time to learn to use the way we pay attention to create a more vibrant reality.

This book will teach you what you need to know to put attention training to work. It explains the Open-Focus system of attention. It includes exercises that will allow you to expand your attention into an Open Focus. It gives you tools to increase your awareness of how you are paying attention and to help you recognize different styles of attention. And it will teach you how to carry a newfound Open-Focus attention from the exercises into everything you do—from work to play to family life—to make your life more effortless and more rewarding.

NOTES ON USING THE AUDIO PROGRAM

Enclosed at the end of this book is an audio CD of guided exercises in which I guide listeners through two fundamental Open-Focus exercises: "Head and Hands," which appears in the text following chapter 4; and "General Open-Focus Training," which does not appear in the text. Once you've read enough of the book to understand the uses of Open-Focus training and the theory that underlies it, I recommend listening to the audio exercises at least twice a day in order to gain the maximum benefits.

In the book I offer additional exercises, geared toward specific types of problems, that are not included on the CD. To do these exercises I recommend having someone read the questions to you slowly (with fifteen-second intervals between the guiding questions) or reading the exercises in this manner into a tape recorder and playing them back to yourself. (The audio CD serves as a model of how subsequent exercises should be read.) To order audio cassettes or CDs of all the Open-Focus exercises, visit www.openfocus.com.

1

An Addiction to Narrow Focus

Attention is the nerve of the whole psychological system.

— EDWARD TITCHENER, PhD,
pioneering attention researcher

SOME DAYS we flow easily through our lives, while other days we struggle to get by. We might feel loving, generous, and absorbed one moment, and critical, unfeeling, or irritable the next. A problem might feel overwhelming in the morning and seem like "no big deal" by afternoon. A pain in a leg may pound one minute and feel like it's gone the next. What accounts for these changes? In my view, the most fundamental reason is a spontaneous change in styles of paying attention. People are affected by shifts in attention all the time, but they usually don't realize that changes in how they feel have to do with changes in the way they attend to thoughts, emotions, and physical sensations.

Shifts in styles of attention—in the way we shape and direct our awareness—play a large, unrecognized role in our lives. In fact, our choice of type and direction of our attention is vital. Certain kinds of attention can quickly dissolve physical pain and emotional stress and can cause widespread changes in physiology. It is my view that any therapy or relaxation technique that helps us make positive changes works, at least in part, by bringing about beneficial shifts in attention.

A large part of the pleasure and relaxation we get from watching a movie or fishing or going on vacation, for example, derives from these activities changing, for a while, the way we pay attention. On vacation we stop narrowly focusing on the bills, work, or other responsibilities, and our physiology responds in a positive way. Vacations also broaden attention to include a multisensory awareness (for example, the whiff of salt water or the smell of pine trees) as we take in uncommon environs we have not yet learned about.

My own research and clinical experience over the past four decades strongly suggest that the way we attend has powerful and immediate effects on the nervous system. (For a detailed scientific overview of my research into the role of attention in mental and physical health, see the appendix and www.open focus.com.)

Attention is all-encompassing in our lives. Feeling at home is the result of a way of paying attention. Love is a way of paying attention. When we pay attention in a rigid, effortful, and thus stressed way, it is a drag on the entire mind-body system: We are more likely to overreact in ways that are fearful, angry, effortful, rigid, and resistant. When we pay attention in a flexible way we are more accepting, comfortable, energetic, aware, healthy, productive, and in the flow. Full attention leads to creativity, spontaneity, acceptance, faith, empathy, integration, productivity, flexibility, efficiency, stress reduction, endurance, persistence, accuracy, perspective, and compassion.

Let me clarify an essential point about improving our health and well-being through the power of our attention: The issue is not *what* we attend to. Far more critical is *how* we attend, *how* we form and direct our awareness, and *how* we adhere—rigidly or flexibly—to a chosen style of attention.

Whether we realize it or not, we pay attention with our whole body and mind, in ways that are measurable. Our style of attention impacts the brain's electrical rhythms, as can be shown in an electroencephalogram, or EEG.

Because the brain is the master control panel for our mind and body, when we change its electrical patterns we initiate systemwide effects, including changes in muscle tension, respiratory rate, and the flow of neurotransmitters and hormones. Our perception, memory, information processing, performance, physiology, and emotional well-being are all influenced by (and, in my view, often subordinate to) attention.

In our culture we do not recognize or make use of the full repertoire of attention styles. Few of us are consciously aware that there are different styles of attention, each with different qualities and each suited to different kinds of tasks. Instead, we are culturally biased to stay locked in limited modes of attention, to our great detriment. Many of my clients feel trapped or walled in, and they do not know what the walls are made of or how to dissolve them. Many know they built the walls themselves somehow, but they think they are constructed out of the content of their awareness—by the things that have happened to them in their lives—or by any number of external factors and their thoughts about them. They can't find their way out because they are stuck in a process of continually scanning the content of their problems for a solution, when the walls that trap them are largely made out of attentional biases.

Prepared for the Hunt

On the African savanna, a pride of lions lie on a grassy rise, half asleep, muscles relaxed, breathing slowly as the warm sun soaks into their backs. When a herd of gazelles wanders into sight, several heads go up. But the real change comes when the lions notice that one of the animals appears to be injured. Suddenly, without moving, they narrow their gaze on that one animal; all else, including the other gazelles, is relegated to the background. They hear only the sound of the bleating gazelle, nothing else. The lions have moved from a relaxed, diffuse form of attention to a more intense, single-pointed, visual focus, and as a result their arousal levels rise: Muscles tense and heart and respiratory rates increase as they prepare for the chase.

I call this style of attention "narrow-objective" attention or focus, and it is how, without realizing it, the vast majority of us pay attention most of the time, to both our internal and external worlds. Narrow-objective attention is focusing on one or a few important things as the foreground, and dismissing all other stimuli, making everything else the background.

As I mentioned earlier, the way we pay attention has a measurable impact on our brain waves, as recorded by an EEG. Using the EEG, scientists have also demonstrated that different styles of attention correspond to particular brain-wave frequencies. Brain-wave activity normally is recorded in the 1–50 hertz range. Hertz (Hz) is a unit of frequency, representing the number of cycles per second: the higher the hertz, the faster the frequency. So-called brain waves are the electrical representations of brain activity. Each cell's electrical activity is summed up, moment by moment, to create composite electrical rhythms that are called brain waves, which can be measured through the scalp and skull.

The range of normal brain-wave frequencies is generally divided into four groups. Delta (0.5–4 hertz), the slowest, is produced during sleep. Theta (4–8 hertz) is produced during twilight consciousness, between feeling deeply relaxed or daydreaming and falling asleep. Alpha (8–12 hertz) is also produced during relaxed states but those in which we are still alert. The active frequencies, or beta (13–50 hertz), are where we carry out most of our tasks. Beta is usually divided into three subgroups: low, mid, and high range. Low beta (13–15 hertz) is characterized by relaxed but interested attention, characteristic of someone taking a test who knows the material

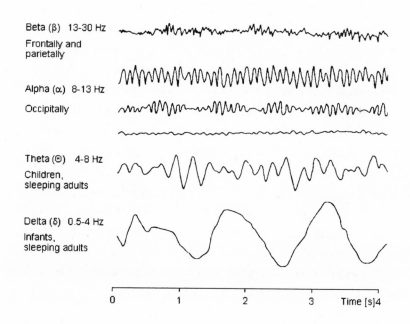

Beta (β) 13-30 Hz
Frontally and
parietally

Alpha (α) 8-13 Hz
Occipitally

Theta (Θ) 4-8 Hz
Children,
sleeping adults

Delta (δ) 0.5-4 Hz
Infants,
sleeping adults

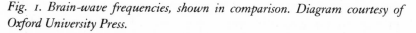

Fig. 1. Brain-wave frequencies, shown in comparison. Diagram courtesy of Oxford University Press.

well. Mid-range beta (16–22 hertz) is produced during focused, external attention. Frequencies of this range and higher are associated with the dominant use of narrow focus. High beta (22 hertz and higher) is often correlated with tense muscles, anger, anxiety, and other intense emotions. Examples include someone taking an important test who doesn't know the material, or someone screaming at another driver because he cut him off. (However, frequencies around 40 Hz have recently been observed in higher quantities in long-term meditators.)

Narrow-objective focus is an emergency mode of paying attention that quickly and substantially increases the frequency of the brain's electrical activity and raises other aspects of physiological arousal, such as heart and respiratory rates, which in turn directly affect our perception, emotions, and behavior. While narrow-objective focus allows us to perform some tasks very well, it is also physiologically and psychologically expensive because chronic use results in the accumulation of stress. It takes a great deal of energy to perpetually maintain this type of attention, even though we usually aren't aware of it. In narrow focus the central nervous system is more inherently unstable and more highly reactive than other modes of attention.

Evolution provided humans with this narrow beam of attention to respond, in the short run, to urgent or important external situations. There's nothing inherently wrong with it; in fact, one reason it is overused is precisely because it is so helpful and allows us, in the short run, to accomplish so much. What's wrong is our near-complete dependence on it and addiction to it.

Not everything is urgent, but we can treat it that way. It's like driving a sports car in one gear all the time. With our foot on the accelerator, motor racing, we spend so much time in this mode that we don't realize we are in it, that we may be doing damage to the transmission, engine, and other parts, or that we can grab the shifter and change our speed. Open-Focus attention training does just that—it demonstrates the other gears of attention, allowing trainees to operate the gearshift and get the best performance out of the car.

CONDITIONED TO NARROW-OBJECTIVE ATTENTION

In our material society, narrow-objective focus is the coin of the realm—and we seldom question it. We adopt it because it pays off, at least in the short run. Our culture affirms personal relationships not by common experiences of oneness or union, but by the sharing and reiteration of common objective experiences, whatever form they take, whether it's a sporting event, a thought or feeling, or a new purchase. People can talk for hours about a football or baseball game, remembering each and every detail, going over it again and again. They talk about the objects they have purchased or want to purchase. Or they chat about movies and television shows. We are rewarded, respected, despised, criticized, loved, punished, accepted, or rejected based upon our ability to focus on, objectify, name, recall, and verbalize our thoughts and experiences. If you can't do it well, you are stigmatized—you can feel left out, alienated, different, or, worse, completely ignored.

We all remember commands like these from childhood and adolescence: "Pay attention to your homework"; "Pay attention to the teacher"; "Stop daydreaming"; "Concentrate"; "Watch where you are going"; "Be careful"; "Look out for cars"; "Keep your eye on the road." What your parents or teacher really meant was that you weren't paying narrow enough attention to them or to what they felt was important, that you weren't doing a good job of excluding everything else, particularly in the external world, from your awareness. You were in fact paying attention, even if it was to something else, in your own way, or to your thoughts and ideas. But the more we mirror the attention strategies of our parents, friends, and other companions, the more we gain their trust and acceptance. There's a lot of pressure for us to adopt narrow-objective attention most of the time.

The number of things that require attention has grown exponentially in modern times, and trying to manage and control all this new experience and information has become an obsession. We live in an object-oriented society, awash, internally and externally, in a sea of sense objects—finite things such as thoughts, sounds, feelings, tastes, smells, and visual images—much, if not all, of the time. In addition, the tasks we have to accomplish at work and at home are long and often complicated. Television bombards us with ads for everything from cars to phones to clothes to diamond rings. Stores are crammed with thousands of objects. We use cell phones and computers and video games and pagers. We follow our favorite bands and download ring tones. We place great value in and survey the broadest array of sense objects in history. There is an unprecedented variety of sense objects available to us and we value sense objects more highly than did people in any other historical periods.

The "information flow" has become a torrent. In their book *The Attention Economy,* Thomas Davenport and John Beck, both leading business strategists, argue that the biggest problem in today's business world is combating what they call "organizational ADD," the difficulty people have knowing what to pay attention to during the course of a typical workday. There are simply too many demands on our attention. One issue of the Sunday *New York Times,* for example, contains more factual information than all of the written material available to readers in the fifteenth century. More than sixty thousand books are published every year in the United States. There are more than two billion Web pages on the Internet, which in over a decade has become as much a part of our lives as television.

We use narrow-objective attention as a way of wading through this flood of information, as an attempt to evaluate it and assign priorities within it. Whatever you think of the benefits of our material and information society, it's obvious that the brain requires a great deal of time and energy to take it all in and sort it all out. Ours is a busy society, and our brains stay busy keeping apace with it. All too often our narrow, rigid attention to the world around us engenders a fatigue that is the source of many of our problems.

ATTENTION AND FEAR

Stress is not just a problem of too much going on. How we attend to our emotions is the critical element of our addiction to narrow-objective focus. Narrow focus occurs when our well-being is threatened—a reflexive response to fearful situations.

Take the case of a boy I'll call Kyle. Each afternoon, as his school bus drew closer to his home, dread grew in the pit of his stomach. Would his father be home? Had he been drinking? His father exploded into rages when he drank; he would hunt Kyle down and whip him with a belt for any transgression, real or imagined. He looked at other kids on the bus laughing and talking. Couldn't he go to someone else's home?

Kyle eventually ended up in foster care, which sent him to a special school for children who had been traumatized. Among other things, abuse and neglect at an early age affect a child's cognitive abilities, and Kyle's teachers realized that he had trouble reading. The problem wasn't that he needed glasses; it was that his field of vision was so small he could only focus on one word at a time and couldn't tell what the next word was. He stumbled and stuttered as he read. Teachers taught him exercises to relax his eye muscles and eventually, as his visual scope broadened, he could see two, then three, words at a time, and finally phrases. Several months later he had learned to read smoothly and confidently.

As a victim of abuse, Kyle suffered from extreme narrow focus, a condition triggered by life in a home that was chaotic and hostile from the day he was born. He could never be sure when or where the next threat would come. Kyle responded to this lack of safety by instinctively becoming hypervigilant in narrow-objective focus, constantly scanning his environment for danger, always apprehensive and fearing attack.

Vision is critical to any animal's survival. However, the eye is extremely susceptible to stress. People who experience chronic stress develop a chronically narrowed visual field, which over the long term impacts eyesight. Our visual system is also hardwired to our emotions. Just as the resting lion reflexively prepares for the hunt when he spies gazelles, human beings respond to external problems, threats, or perceived threats by heightening their arousal and narrowing their gaze.

While Kyle's case is extreme, almost everyone suffers from chronic narrow focus to some degree, predominantly due to emotional stress and extreme focus. Much stress originates in childhood, when we are too inexperienced to understand the world. Taking tests when we don't know the material, being threatened by a bully, or (especially) feeling that our parents don't love us—whether or not this is true—are a few of the things that condition us to narrow focus.

Chronic narrow-objective focus creates a behavioral loop. Narrow focus exacerbates fearful circumstances; and then when circumstances have changed and we are no longer in "danger," we tend to stay in narrow focus as a way of avoiding our residual feelings of fear and anxiety, accompanied by a middle- to high-beta range of frequencies to keep unpleasant feelings from surfacing.

In this sense, narrow focus is used as a strategy to escape. As feelings of anxiety rise we unconsciously look for effective distractions to keep us from feeling them. We rivet attention on an engrossing novel or fast-paced television show or thrilling video game in part to escape emotional chaos, anxiousness, or unpleasantness from within. The more interested we are in something "out there," the more effective it is as an anxiety-management technique.

The power of using narrow focus for diversion is being researched at the University of Washington Harborview Burn Treatment Center. For people who have been severely burned, peeling off old bandages is extremely painful. Even morphine can only dull, not eliminate, the excruciating pain. Researchers here placed two subjects who were undergoing wound care in a virtual reality environment. In one part of the study, each played a standard video game on a television during the process of bandage removal. In the other part they wore goggles and traveled through an immersive virtual world and played a game where they had to shoot snowballs at attackers. One patient thought of his pain 95 percent of the time while playing the video game but just 2 percent of the time while his attention was diverted by his actions in virtual reality. The other patient went from thinking of his pain 91 percent of the time to 36 percent in virtual reality. "Conscious attention is like a spotlight," one of the researchers said. "With virtual reality we attract the spotlight to the virtual world and away from the pain."[1]

In fact, without realizing it, many of us use our attention to manage our physical and emotional pain. The more successfully our attention is diverted, the less pain we feel. At some point, however, pain and anxiety become so great that diversionary tactics don't work. Think back to my unsuccessful effort to distract my attention away from the intense kidney-stone pain by bending my thumb or pinching myself. If attention diversion works, we'll keep using it until it stops being effective or becomes too expensive. When it stops working we'll find something more potent. Diversionary strategies are often overused to the point of addiction; compulsive use of television, food, sex, gambling, travel, video games, loud music, alcohol, drugs, and especially work can all serve as strategic distractions to keep us away from—or help us manage—our pain.

People even use this strategy as they fall asleep, because the emotional tones of past events have a tendency to surface as we relax and drift into sleep. Staying in narrow focus is one way of keeping the brain distracted and thus preventing us from remembering painful memories. I have clients who cannot fall asleep without a loud radio or TV playing—they need music or talk shows or other external stimuli to divert their attention from the feeling of memories that arise in the theta state on the edge of sleep.

The effort it takes to chronically divert the mind from these feelings causes the accumulation of tension and leads to fatigue and burnout, and depression can be the end result.

However, at the same time, because we live in a culture that rewards it, narrow-objective attention can serve us well much of the time: We get good grades, drive carefully, feel accepted, and learn to operate safely and productively in a busy, demanding world. We don't recognize paying attention effortfully and chronically as a problem. Some people may never notice the problems it causes. Chronic narrow-objective attention requires a great deal of energy and, in my view, keeps us from knowing our true selves. Yet most of us aren't aware of the tension that the use of chronic narrow focus produces. We've become habituated to it. But maintaining a tense, emergency mode of attention tires us out; and so we need another cup of coffee to muster the energy to keep paying attention, or a cigarette or a glass of wine to relieve the tension of narrow focus.

Chronic narrow-objective attention ultimately prevents the diffusion of stress. Even in a life that is relatively carefree by current standards, stress can and does accumulate to levels that produce symptoms of disorder and disease (though we often don't recognize them as being caused by stress). Preventing the diffusion of stress and causing its accumulation, narrow-objective focus actually makes us less productive over the long haul. People who complain of an inability to concentrate, listlessness, low productivity, diminished sexual activity, and depression often find these problems resolved when they learn to shift out of narrow-objective attention.

On a psychological level, when we remain in narrow-objective focus, fear and anxiety play an exaggerated role in our minds and adversely color our perceptions of the world around us. Though we may not realize it, narrow-objective focus and the resultant stress that we bottle up inside keep us emotionally numb, blocking many feelings from our awareness. We miss out on rich experiences of smell and taste, pleasant physical sensations, and deep feelings of joy and sadness. Ironically, and tragically, although this constant narrow-objective focus is how we attempt to connect emotionally with other people, and with experience itself, it is exactly the wrong way for making these kinds of connections.

Objectifying things or people in emergency mode reduces empathy and distances us from experience, creating feelings of separation. That's why people so often feel isolated or thwarted

23

in their relationships, or feel that their experiences are not deep or meaningful. They often seek out the stimulation of new relationships and experiences instead. There is nothing wrong with them, but there is something wrong with how rigidly they attend. Satisfying unions, whether with other people or with our own internal experiences, are much easier when attention is flexible, when narrow and objective forms of attention give way easily to other, more relaxed, diffuse, and immersed styles of attention. And although some of us already may have caring relationships in narrow-objective attention, these can be enhanced by learning the attentional flexibility that comes with Open-Focus training.

Exercise

Expanding Your Awareness
of Visual Space

To PROVIDE a glimpse of how things in everyday life change as you change the way you pay attention, try the following exercise. As you continue to read this page, allow yourself to be aware of the three-dimensional physical space between your eyes and the words printed on the page. Let the awareness occur gradually as you continue reading. Because we are conditioned to sense only objects and exclude space, it may take some time for you to become aware of this visual sensation of physical space. Once you do become aware of the space, pause for a few seconds as you gently maintain that awareness.

Now, without shifting your eyes from the page, gradually begin to sense the space that is to the right and to the left of the page. Let your peripheral field of vision widen spontaneously at its own pace to take in that awareness. And once you develop that awareness, enjoy it for a few seconds.

Now allow your visual background to come forward, to become as important as your visual foreground. In other words, the whole page, the edges of the book, the table and walls behind the book, can be made foreground simultaneously with the words you are reading. This, too, should be carried out effortlessly and naturally. It may seem difficult at first, but it is well within our capacity to focus in this way. Sit for a few seconds as you gently maintain this awareness, and allowing background and foreground to become equally important or interesting.

As you continue reading, also include the appearance of space that surrounds your entire body. Allow time for this perception to take place as your visual awareness opens and broadens into three dimensions. Now permit yourself to become aware of the space between the lines you are reading, even as you continue to read. Also bring into your awareness the space between the words themselves, and then the space between the letters of the words. Your awareness of visual space can continue to expand effortlessly while your awareness of letters, words, and concepts continues.

Expanding your three-dimensional visual awareness of space is creating a change in the way you are paying attention. You may also begin to sense your awareness expanding into other sensations of the absence we call space—feeling it, tasting and smelling it, hearing silence, experiencing the space and silence in your mind from which visual images and internal dialogue emerge, along with a limitless sense of now.

As you continue to allow your awareness to open and become more inclusive, you may notice subtle alterations in your reading experience. Your understanding of what you are reading may become more centered, enriched, and engaged. It may become easier to read the words. Thoughts of things unrelated to what you are reading may float effortlessly through your mind. Perhaps your eyes feel less strained as you read. Perhaps your hand supporting the book feels more relaxed. Breathing may come more easily. You may discover that muscles in your face or neck have started to loosen somewhat or that your position in the chair has become more comfortable. You may feel more whole or unified. You may also feel rising up some mildly unpleasant feelings that have been repressed by the sustained act of narrow focusing. The process of dissolving these unpleasant feelings will be described in a later chapter.

If you notice even small changes during the reading exercises, you have begun to experience some of the benefits of Open Focus. It may seem strange, even uncomfortable at first, for we all have learned to pay narrow and effortful attention to what we read and to most other things. Narrow-objective focus is thought to be necessary to resist distractions so that we can understand, analyze, and do something about what we read. That idea is so ingrained that many of us have become unaware of the mental and physical stress and fatigue that accompany this constant gripping. Our eyes grip the words, our minds grip the concepts, while our fingers may literally clutch the book. But we don't need this level of effort merely for reading. By comparison, Open Focus releases effortful attention and allows us to spend just the right amount of effort, rather than chronically overdoing it. A precise, relaxed, yet interested attention—a lightly held narrow-objective attention amid a diffuse immersed background of space—is maintained, while tension and stress diffuse and dissolve.

This exercise can be used while doing almost anything, from riding the subway to talking on the telephone to cooking to working on the computer. Stopping what you are doing and becoming aware of your peripheral vision of space and the space between you and the objects around you is a way to begin incorporating Open Focus into everyday life.

Sweet Surrender

DISCOVERING THE BENEFITS OF SYNCHRONOUS ALPHA BRAIN WAVES

A Zen student once asked his teacher Ikkyu,
a fifteenth-century Zen master, to sum up
the highest wisdom. The master responded
to this enormous question with a single
word scratched in the sand: "Attention."
The student wasn't satisfied and asked him
to elaborate. Ikkyu wrote, "Attention.
Attention. Attention."

I STARTED to formulate my ideas about attention when I was an assistant professor of psychology at the State University of New York at Stony Brook in the late 1960s. My initial research had nothing to do with helping people to relax or feel better. As a graduate student at UCLA, I had researched visual perception in macaque monkeys and found that a fundamental principle of how the brain communicates with itself is something called synchrony—when the brain's electrical activity, or brain waves, are synchronized in one or more areas of the brain.[1] The greater the ability to enter into and exit synchrony in brain-wave activity, the better the brain performs its tasks. This is true no matter what the frequency. Over the course of a day, our brains naturally move in and out of synchrony, but we can actually train ourselves to achieve greater control of synchrony.

At SUNY Stony Brook I wanted to study the role of synchrony in the human nervous system to see if it would lead to greater subtlety, clarity, speed, and scope of information processing and perception. Since synchronous activity is most prominent when the brain is in a relaxed but alert state, I needed to find a way for human subjects to enhance this activity. Early research had proven that people could control their brain's electrical activity with the help of feedback. But as I experimented on myself, I realized I was on to something more important than just the study of synchrony.

Commercial EEG-biofeedback instruments weren't available in 1967, so I designed and built my own. Connected to a pen-and-ink EEG and an oscilloscope, in a soundproof room, I sat upright in a comfortable chair. A sensor was attached just above the inion (the bump on the back of the head). During twelve two-hour sessions over the course of the next four weeks I struggled in every way imaginable to produce alpha waves (8–12 Hz). I tried with eyes closed and tried with eyes open. I filled the room with negative ions, incense, music, and different colored lights. None seemed to create much alpha. Finally, in the thirteenth session, I was exasperated and gave up and accepted the fact that it was simply impossible for me to create more than baseline alpha on demand. Fortunately I was still connected when I gave up. The second I deeply accepted my failure, the EEG registered high-amplitude alpha production, five times the amplitude and abundance I had been producing before. I got rhythm! I couldn't believe it. I had been trying too hard and didn't know it. By surrendering I had slipped into alpha—the alert, wakeful relaxation that had eluded me. Even though I had learned you couldn't control it, at least not force it, I still wanted to, and every time I tried to produce it I was frustrated and couldn't.

As my experiment continued, I found that I could increase the duration and amplitude, or power, of my alpha. After a few hours in alpha some curious and wonderful changes started to happen. My muscle tone softened, and I moved with a newfound effortlessness and fluidity; sometimes I felt like I was gliding when I walked. Anxiety evaporated. I felt extraordinarily present, centered, poised, open, lighter and freer, more calmly energetic and spontaneous. I laughed and smiled more. Untoward events no longer threw me the way they had before. Arthritic pain in my joints subsided. My senses improved, vision and hearing foremost among them. Colors were more vibrant. I could pick up the subtle scent of perfume long after someone had walked down a hallway. I not only heard sounds I hadn't noticed before but also became more aware of the silence in which the sounds occurred. My obsessive-compulsive style mellowed, and I taught complex graduate-level courses with newfound ease. Friends and family responded positively. I was more aware of the bigger picture. Yet I didn't feel as if I had lost my edge; indeed, the things I had been doing—teaching and researching—came easier and more clearly than before.

I was in the zone. There was a feeling that I had come home after a long absence, home to who I really was. The feeling lasted for many months, and with more training it could be refreshed. I felt strongly that this is the way life was meant to be.

And from an evolutionary point of view it made a great deal of sense. Chronic depression, anxiety, and a host of other physical and psychological problems are not the natural state of human beings. Nor are they necessarily the result of a brain that is somehow fundamentally flawed. Instead they are the result of "operator error." Alpha isn't magical—it just seems that way because we've forgotten how to access it, increase its amplitude, and prolong it. When someone learns to operate their central nervous system the way it was designed to be operated, however, and includes abundant low-frequency synchrony, things run more smoothly and efficiently and don't break down as often. We are equipped with a rapid and sensitive emergency response to assure survival. But we are also equipped with a process of restoration and recovery, a way to lay down our burden: by generating low-frequency synchrony.

The Lesson of Biofeedback

I wasn't the first to discover the power of alpha. That distinction belongs to Dr. Joe Kamiya, a now-retired professor of psychology from the U. C. San Francisco's Langley Porter Psychiatric Institute and a friend. In 1965 he was researching the ability of people to recognize what frequency range their brain was in. Kamiya wired each student volunteer to an EEG; and as the student lay in a darkened chamber, the professor spoke to him by intercom and watched as the young man's EEG tracings were scribbled on paper. "Keep your eyes closed," Kamiya told him softly. "Listen to a series of tones. After each tone sounded, the subject was to guess if he felt he was producing a particular brain wave that Kamiya was watching for on the EEG recorder. That was all the information the student would get. By watching the tracings of the EEG, Kamiya knew if it was alpha being produced, but the subject did not. When the subject said "yes" or "no," Kamiya would answer "correct" if he was in alpha or "wrong" if he wasn't.

During the first session the subject seemed to be guessing. But by the third and fourth sessions he could easily tell when he was in alpha almost every time. By the fourth session the young man correctly guessed his brain state four hundred times in a row. The experiment ended only when the subject thought he was being tricked with so many "yes" answers and purposely gave the wrong answer. Kamiya was flabbergasted that the young man could recognize his EEG frequency so successfully.

Following up, Kamiya wanted to see if the student could generate alpha at will. "Go into the alpha state when you hear a bell ring once," the young man was told. "If it rings twice do not go into alpha." The student was perfect. Over the next few months he and others demonstrated adroit control over their brain waves.

What would later capture the public's imagination about Kamiya's work, however, was not the fact that people could learn to control their EEG, but the benefits some subjects claimed after they spent hours generating alpha: They felt refreshed, clear, relaxed, and centered in a way they had never experienced before. Colors took on a new richness and the world seemed fresher. They felt less depressed and less anxious. It was a eureka moment for Kamiya. "Instead of gulping a tranquilizer," he wrote in a 1968 *Psychology Today* article about the experiments, "one might merely reproduce the state of tranquillity that he learned with the kind of training used in our studies."

Kamiya's article led to a tremendous outpouring of interest in EEG biofeedback, with many proclaiming it a shortcut to enlightenment that would transform society. Other researchers built their own biofeedback technologies and manufacturers rushed equipment—much of it flawed—to market. The hype, however, got ahead of the science and many of the claims made by some manufacturers and researchers were exaggerated. Meanwhile, other researchers, who wanted to debunk these claims, used faulty methodologies in their studies or simply denounced the benefits of alpha training without evidence. But the response people had to generating alpha was a very real phenomenon, and many subsequent studies showed that.[2] Unfortunately, in part because of too many exaggerated claims, these later studies were largely ignored.

The transcendent experiences of Kamiya's students corresponded precisely to what I had experienced. But there was one other change I noticed. In addition to those feelings, I noticed that the brain-wave training broadened my attention; I took in the world visually in a very different way. I now perceived larger scenes without focusing on any one element and with much less effort. I went back to some of the writings of Hans Berger, who discovered the existence of the brain's electrical output and who, in the 1930s, reported on the association between alpha and a state of relaxed attentiveness. But it wasn't just visual. My awareness of the room I was in, my feeling and sense of it, was also much bigger. It was my first inkling of Open-Focus attention.

So, at the time, two critical discoveries had emerged. First, it dawned on me that producing alpha caused my attention to shift from narrow to diffuse, thus opening my awareness. Second, I realized that subjects could relax and produce abundant alpha not only with eyes-closed biofeedback but also by changing the way they paid attention in an eyes-open state. Changing the way they paid attention manifested in the EEG. And when they attended in full Open Focus, they not only produced alpha, but a very specific kind called phase-synchronous alpha.

Phase synchrony means not only that many parts of the brain are producing alpha but that these waves are also rising and falling in unison. This means that a large number of cells are working together—an especially powerful type of synergistic cortical activity. While high-frequency, nonsynchronous beta activity is like the chatter of an auditorium full of high school students engaged in separate conversations, the synchronized, uniform lower frequency generated across the whole brain by open styles of attention is the equivalent of the same group of students singing together.[3]

Though it is made only of light, a laser beam is powerful enough to use as a cutting torch because the light waves are in phase. Dr. William Tiller, professor emeritus of engineering at Stanford University, writes: "If we could somehow take the same number of photons emitted by [a 60-watt] lightbulb per second and orchestrate their emission to be in phase with each other ... the energy density at the surface of the lightbulb would be thousands to millions of times higher than the present photon energy density at the surface of the sun."[4] Soldiers marching in lockstep are in phase synchrony; this phenomenon is so powerful that soldiers have to break cadence when they cross a bridge or they can destroy it. And, although less visibly dramatic than these effects, learning to create phase-synchronous alpha brain waves is an extremely efficient way to release stress.

Once I had recognized the tremendous potential of synchronous alpha, the focus of my research became finding a way to help others produce those brain waves as quickly as possible. It had taken me twelve two-hour sessions before I was able to let go during the thirteenth session and increase alpha amplitude and duration. That was simply too long, and many people would give up before they experienced the release. And it defies verbal instruction. The only way it could be learned efficiently was through experience.

Much Ado about Nothing

Nothing is more real than nothing.

—Samuel Beckett

In 1971 I discovered a shortcut. In research experiments student volunteers were exposed to a number of relaxation methods as their EEG was monitored to see which exercises produced the most phase-synchronous alpha. Some were asked to visualize peaceful scenes and locations. Some listened to their favorite music. Others tried fragrances, negative-ion generation, and colored lights. Some of these things had a mild alpha-enhancing effect; most had very little impact. One day I tried a standard twenty-item relaxation inventory. During the first few questions—imagine a dewdrop on a rose petal or a cascading waterfall, for example—their EEG manifested little change. Then I asked. "Can you imagine the space between your eyes?" Boom. The pens scribbled the symmetrical waves of high-amplitude alpha. A subsequent question was, "Can you imagine the space between your ears?" Again, boom, high-amplitude alpha appeared instantly. When either of these "space"-related questions was asked, subjects almost invariably generated a significant increase in alpha brain synchrony in the brain sites being monitored. No other question or imagery brought about such profound changes in the EEG. "Objectless imagery"—the multisensory experience and awareness of space, nothingness, or absence—almost always elicits large amplitude and prolonged periods of phase-synchronous alpha activity.

"Nothing" is not merely nothing. Nothing, in fact, is a great and robust healer and is critical to the health and well-being of our nervous system. Space is unique among the contents of attention because space, silence, and timelessness cannot be concentrated on or grasped as a separate experience. It slips through, permeates your attention, through all your senses. Seeing, hearing, tasting, feeling, smelling, and thinking of space, basking in it—while simultaneously experiencing timelessness—is a powerful way to let go, the most powerful way that I know.

Simply by watching EEG activity, I discovered the robust effects of the awareness of space on the central nervous system in my own way. But I was certainly not the first to realize that being aware of space or nothing has value. I've since found other examples of perceiving space and nothingness as a goal of meditation. One Eastern mystic wrote that it was important to "attain a state of mind in which even though surrounded by crowds of people, it is as if you were alone in a field extending for tens of thousands of miles." The Japanese have a philosophy of *ma*—the ability to see the space between objects as well as the objects themselves. Other traditions use guided visual meditations on mandalas, in which practitioners focus on the space between the lines of the sacred symbols. All of these "technologies" no doubt slow cortical rhythms and relax the central nervous system; certainly they deserve further study and research.

Indeed, work by several researchers would later show that phase-synchronous alpha is the hallmark of veteran meditators.[5] What I'd done, in effect, was to discover some of the Western correlates of Eastern spiritual disciplines and describe them in the language of psychology and physiology.

Since a sustained awareness of space is key to Open-Focus attention, I recorded a series of exercises to guide people through different kinds of objectless imagery, asking them to imagine space first between and around body regions and then through them, extending limitlessly in every direction. For example, I ask listeners to imagine space in, around, and through their eyes, neck, head, and hands (which leads to a release of those areas) and ultimately space extending limitlessly in every direction. When people gently direct their awareness to it and imagine feeling space, the brain responds immediately, dropping into whole-brain synchronous alpha. Connected to instruments that show them when they are in synchronous alpha, subjects can learn to change very quickly; some notice positive changes in mood, tension, and anxiety—all widely reported effects of alpha—in a single half-hour session.[6] And long-term effects included improved memory, clearer thinking, and heightened creativity.[7]

What is the physiological mechanism underlying the sudden and powerful effect on the brain of imagining space, silence, and timelessness? Part of it may be that the brain is very active when it is making sense out of the world. When it is processing sense objects—either physical or imagined—it uses high-frequency, desynchronized beta activity in order to make that processing possible. Electrical signals move through the brain at speeds exceeding a hundred miles an hour in many different and disparate regions. For example, research at Princeton University on monkeys found that when the eyes of the animal locate an object not only do the visual centers get busy, but there is also activity elsewhere. Neurons rapidly fire in the ventral premotor cortex, which coordinates muscle activity with what the animal sees, hears, and feels, a firing that continues well after the object is gone. In fact, the parts of the brain responsible for sense perception and voluntary action become activated when we simply *imagine* objects and actions. EEG research shows that when athletes imagine performing their sport, for example, the brain activates in the same regions as when they are actually performing.[8]

When the mind is asked to imagine or attend to space, however, there is nothing—no-*thing*—to grip on to, to objectify and make sense of, no memories of past events or anticipation of future scenarios. The brain is allowed to take a vacation. This is presumably why cortical rhythms slow quickly into alpha, and later into theta, and the same brain that was racing moments before becomes a stress-reducing brain and a quiet mind. The imagination and realization of space seems to reset stress-encumbered neural networks and return them to their original effortlessly flexible processing. Then, after this "vacation," overall performance is enhanced.

Even as it relaxes the brain's attention mechanisms, imagining space opens the scope of attention very quickly. And while imagining space most prominently affects our vision, it opens the other senses as well. In fact, just closing one's eyes causes a prominent increase of synchronous alpha over the whole brain, not only in the visual system. This suggests that synchrony's role is a more general and fundamental one, like attention.

In my experience, objectless imagery is the quickest way to get into an open focus, and an awareness of space is a powerful tool to teach people to access and maintain alternative styles of attention. We can also transfer this awareness of space to everyday life. Moreover, if we pay attention to stress in an open style as it occurs, it doesn't accumulate and stay bottled up; it is immediately experienced and released to go through on its merry way. If we are not only aware of the things around us, but also admit an awareness of space, silence, and a sense of timelessness as the ground of our experience, we have the ability to lead a much less stressful life.

When we are fully capable of flexible attention, we can readily move into alternative forms of brain activity when emergency functions aren't needed, just as the lioness does after the hunt. Presumably the lioness that fixes on a single object of prey, one gazelle among a herd, chases and brings down the animal in narrow-objective attention. During the hunt the targeted gazelle was foreground, and all other gazelles besides the chosen one were rendered peripheral background—even though they might be physically closer. Narrow focus played its role—it induced a surge of adrenaline, increased blood flow to the large muscle groups, and increased heart rate to support stalking, chasing, and the takedown.

When the chase ends, the lioness's attention moves out of narrow focus and increases diffuse attention where there is no longer a strong distinction between figure and ground. If the herd of gazelles remains, the lioness now sees all of them, as well as the other elements of the landscape, equally. It is an attentional shift away from emergency function. The sympathetic nervous system quiets and parasympathetic function increases. The lioness moves toward a multisensory awareness, feeling the sun on her back again and aware of the scents and sounds around her. Muscles relax, hormonal flows adjust, and blood flow is redistributed. The body normalizes.

The physiological and mental recovery that occurs with whole-brain synchrony and its attentional correlates is the basis for the clinical approach that I have used with clients for the last thirty years.

3

The Full
Complement
of Attention

Petite, attractive, and energetic with dark blond hair, Paula was a charge nurse who worked round-the-clock shifts caring for heart patients in a postcoronary care unit at a major medical center. It was a demanding job, with life-or-death outcomes, and its effects on her were exacerbated by a naturally intense personality. Clearly worn out by her circumstances, she came to the Princeton Biofeedback Center, flopped into a chair, and complained of a number of seemingly unrelated symptoms—bouts of anxiety, frequent and debilitating headaches, constant stomach pains, endometriosis, mild depression, and insomnia. A doctor had prescribed various medications, she told me, but she balked, not wanting to mask her symptoms with drugs or risk the possible side effects associated with the long-term use of medication. She primarily hoped to treat her anxiety, the most uncomfortable of her symptoms.

For Paula there was no talk therapy prescribed and she refused medications; instead, for several weeks, twice a week, she learned one overriding lesson: to change the way she paid attention. For twenty-five to forty-five minutes Paula listened to recorded Open-Focus exercises that asked her to close her eyes and gently asked if she could imagine all manner of space—sometimes around her, other times inside her body, other times through her body, extending infinitely in all directions.

Along with the exercises, neurofeedback instruments rewarded her with soft beeps and low-intensity strobe-light flashes when her EEG brain activity reached above threshold levels of synchrony. When the feedback was produced she was moving out of an exclusive narrow-objective attention and toward a diffuse yet still interested style of inclusive attention.

Outside of the clinic, instead of "gripping" the world with a narrow-focused objective attention, she also learned to broaden her field of attention, shifting from a solely narrow-objective focus toward a broader, more inclusive, immersed style of attention.

We treated her anxiety, but we also did a great deal more, for as treatment progressed she realized her problems weren't a bundle of separate symptoms, triggered separately. They had a common cause—the lifelong accumulation of stress enabled by chronic narrow-objective focus, stress that had built up gradually until it produced symptoms of such intensity that she could no longer ignore them.

The simple act of moving out of narrow-objective focus is like relaxing a fist that has been clenched for years. A cascade of changes took place in Paula as she changed the way she attended over the next few weeks. She noticed that the sometimes manic speed of her inner dialogue—the "strategic mind"—slowed considerably. Muscles she had unwittingly been holding tense for years began to relax. Her face, eye, throat, shoulder, and neck muscles in particular began to soften; for these are all muscles that support gripping the world with narrow-objective attention. Color returned to her face. Tension headaches became rare, and her migraines were virtually eliminated. Chronic pain from a spastic colon and endometriosis all but vanished. Her personality softened. After several sessions she described herself as much more at ease and centered. "I can't believe how my life has changed," she said after a few months. "Every single thing in my life was affected for the better."

Changing the way Paula attended to the world didn't, as she had been concerned it might, diminish her ability to work hard or drive or study; in fact those things came easier and she performed them better. Most important, she learned the skills to maintain Open Focus. She learned the difference between a rigidly held narrow focus and a lightly held one. Her newfound flexible attention allowed her to narrow her focus and respond alertly when she needed; but it also taught her to diffuse her attention when she didn't need to concentrate so intently, which gave her the ability to manage her stress load. She learned that both narrow and diffuse attention could simultaneously be present. She learned to transfer her awareness of space to her everyday life; whether helping a patient walk down the hall or eating lunch, she became able to automatically stay aware of space. She learned a fundamental lesson: The way we attend controls the intensity of our experiences and reactions. Narrow focus amplifies the intensity while diffuse focus dilutes it.

Flexible attention is the sine qua non of health.

MOVING OUT OF EMERGENCY MODE

It may seem incredible to believe that so many problems can be alleviated by changing attention style, but it is true. There is an innate and robust normalizing mechanism in the human body, accessed and operated by how we pay attention. I've seen it again and again with my clients. Things they never imagined were caused or exacerbated by stress were resolved with Open-Focus training. And this resolution comes about because narrow-objective focus is an emergency mode of attention.

When we narrow focus we engage our fight-or-flight response, which tamps down some physiological systems that aren't needed for an emergency—immune and digestive functions, for example, get put on the back burner—and ramps up others that are needed, such as muscle tone, quickness of mind, and heart and respiratory rates. That's why stress can lead to digestive problems such as acid-reflux disease and irritable bowel syndrome. Facial pallor is associated with emergency because blood is being shunted away from the skin—that's why stress can lead to dermatological problems. That's the mechanism for pallor, but when stress causes acne it's because high cortisol blood levels cause additional oil secretion, which blocks pores. Also, rashes can be caused by stress when it triggers autoimmune reactions with skin as the target organ. Large muscles become more highly toned during an emergency, preparing us for an attack or an escape, and so chronic narrow-objective attention causes chronic muscle pain. Emergencies slow introspection and induce externally oriented, narrow attention, scanning the environment. And because blood flow is reduced in the frontal lobes of the brain during the stress response, executive functions such as thinking become reactive rather than penetrating and deductive; as a result, one's ability to exercise good judgment and pay appropriate and effective attention is hampered. This explains, in part, why there is such an epidemic of attention deficit disorder (ADD) and attention-deficit/hyperactivity disorder (ADHD).

The stress response is powerful. It's seen in the example of people who do seemingly superhuman things during emergencies, such as lifting a car or moving a rock to free a person pinned beneath. The human body triggers a complex cascade of hundreds of stress chemicals that invade and fortify every organ and muscle of the body. The problem comes when no release of stress follows this surge of preparation; held unabated, the stress response changes our physiology. This is what happens to us when we can't react to or escape from a fearful or threatening situation. While some of this stress dissipates, much of it lingers in our body. Stress isn't necessarily a bad thing—it can be a force that causes us to change and grow. Stress is only a negative if it is unrelenting, prolonged, and accumulating.

Fortunately, stress is not a done deal. It's better thought of as a force that strains our body and mind. Open Focus is a normalizing process, a way of reversing the strains of stress; it allows all systems to return to homeostasis. Stress causes functional, rather than structural, problems; but if it is left to accumulate long enough, its effects can become structural: For example, the brain's hippocampus is reduced in volume in people with untreated depression. As we move into Open Focus the entire central nervous system starts to move out of emergency mode and recover from stress. The brain's electrical activity drops from beta, in the 15 to 45 hertz range, to the more relaxed lower frequencies of 5–15 hertz, a range that encompasses theta, alpha, and the sensory-motor rhythm (SMR). The sympathetic autonomic nervous system, which engages fight or flight, quiets and the parasympathetic autonomic nervous system increases its dominance. Blood flow increases again into the many parts of the body where it had been diminished, bringing them back online, healing them, and improving their function. Different parts of the brain are stimulated by changed blood flow, and neural patterns in the brain shift. Thinking becomes less strategic and more reasoned. There is less generalized fearfulness and anxiety. It becomes easier to sustain attention. Sleep comes more easily. Muscles—from our eye and face muscles to the heart, lungs, and large peripheral muscle groups—enjoy increased blood flow and become more relaxed and less tense. The longer we dwell in this open-attention realm, the more the body is allowed to recover and the more healing takes place. That is, stress diffuses as Open Focus expands.

Once we become aware that there is more than one way to pay attention and learn through Open-Focus training to access these styles of attention, the next step is to transfer our new skills to everyday life. We can learn to do this in every situation—Open-Focus training gives us unparalleled skills and tools to encounter the world in an attentionally flexible way and to effectively manage our reality. Accumulated stress dissolves when one is in Open Focus, and recovery is able to take place continuously as new stress occurs. It becomes second nature to dissolve pain and unwanted experience.

It's not as difficult as it might seem. Everyone learns to ride a bike this way—you pay narrow attention to the many things you need to do—steering, pedaling, and balancing. If you maintain this narrow focus, however, you will run into a tree. Somehow we learn as children to broaden our awareness and bring all these tasks together. Before we know it we're cruising down the street, exhilarated, experiencing a newfound sense of freedom.

STYLES OF ATTENTION

Learning how to move out of the emergency mode of narrow-objective attention and into the relaxed, alert attention of Open Focus is a crucial skill. Open Focus itself is unbiased—that is, it doesn't favor any one style but supports the full range of possible attention styles, which can be present simultaneously. Within Open Focus four main types of attention are possible —*diffuse*, *narrow*, *objective,* and *immersed*—all of which may occur more or less equally and simultaneously. (These don't necessarily exhaust the attention repertoire but are the distinct forms I have identified.) Each style of attention is unique and, when it is emphasized, has significant and different impacts on our physiology, moods, and behavior. Each of the physiological mechanisms that support the different kinds of attention are separate and independent, which means the styles can—and do—exist alone, in combination with others, or all simultaneously.

Figure 2 diagrams the relationship among these types of attention as well as their possible combinations with one another. Each of the four intersecting lines represents a continuum of attention styles, each from zero (at these intersections) to increased levels as the line moves outward.[1]

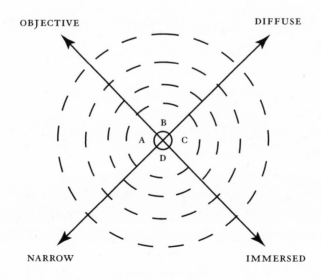

Fig. 2. The Dimensions of Attention: An Objective Model

In *narrow* attention, we can concentrate our attention on a limited field of experience, excluding peripheral perceptions from our awareness. Narrow focus isn't just a way of attending to visual stimuli. We can chronically narrow focus on any sensation, thought, or problem, to the exclusion of almost everything else. For instance, if we are having a conversation while in narrow focus, we are likely to block out sensory input other than the words being spoken and our own private self-talk. As a result, our physical reactions to the content of the conversation can remain inaccessible to our attention. This lack of awareness deprives us of much of our "emotional intelligence" and is especially detrimental when our conversation requires authentic engagement with the other person. In fact, research studies have found that awareness of the physical sensations related to one's problems makes a decisive difference in the success or failure of psychotherapy.[2]

Conversely, in the midst of an argument, we may find ourselves narrowly focusing on angry feelings and a sense of being wronged by the other party. In this case, we may not allow ourselves to listen to the other person or to access thoughts and memories that could help to end the fight and preserve the relationship. In both cases, narrow focus constrains the scope of our attention in a way that does not serve our interests.

Another type of attention is *diffuse* focus, which gives a softer, more inclusive view of the world. Think of attention as the beam of a flashlight. On a camping trip someone might hear a bear cub in a tree. Adjust the light so the beam is narrow, and nearly all of the light will focus on the bear. But if we don't know which tree the animal is in, we can broaden the scope of the flashlight beam so it illuminates more of the forest—including the bear—rather than just one tree.

Diffuse focus is panoramic rather than exclusive or single-pointed; in its most extreme form it is inclusive and three-dimensional, giving equal attention to all internal and external stimuli simultaneously as well as the space, silence, and timelessness in which they occur. No particular target of attention stands out, and the distinctions between figure and ground are blurred or erased. Walking through the forest and being simultaneously aware of the sound of birds singing, the smell of flowers, the feel of a breeze, the view of the trees, and the space and the silence in which these sensory experiences occur is diffuse focus.

The inclusion of both narrow and diffuse attention and their balance is appropriate for most daily life situations. Whereas narrow focus concentrates and intensifies awareness and diffuse focus spreads and moderates experience and reactivity, Open Focus is an inclusive style of attention that admits both narrow and diffuse forms of attention into awareness at the same time. If, while attending in narrow focus, we simply include some awareness of space and of other sense experiences, our attention will be distributed more evenly and our attention will diffuse and dissolve stress.

It's like opening a door from within a darkened room. Just opening the door a crack may permit enough light in the room so that many objects previously in darkness can now be seen. In addition, some air may enter the room, making it easier to breathe. Opening our focus works the same way as opening the door. A little opening can change our perceptual and physical environment significantly.[3]

The axes in figure 2, which run from zero to increased objective attention, relates to the sense of distance or closeness we have to our experience. Flexibility along this continuum is as important to our health and functioning as being able to diffuse and narrow our focus as needed.

Objective attention distances the observer from the object of

49

awareness, enhancing one's conscious ability to evaluate and control it. Different styles of attention are associated with, and supported by, particular body postures and facial expressions. Rodin's sculpture *The Thinker* captures the quintessential posture of objective attention, and you can usually tell when people are increasing this style by their cold or judgmental expression and facial pallor.[4]

Objective attention has allowed humans to step back from the sense of unity that our early ancestors had with the physical world and to discover the laws of nature. This has given rise to innovations that improve our lives in innumerable ways. Unfortunately, it has also alienated us from an awareness that we are a part of nature, which perhaps accounts for our failure to be responsible stewards of the environment.

The last axis in figure 2 relates to *immersed,* or *absorbed,* attention and is characteristic of someone who enters into union with an object or process to the point of self-forgetfulness or unconsciousness. It usually—but not always—has pleasurable connotations. Common examples include the savoring of tastes and the experience of sexual pleasure. People attending in an immersed way usually have an enraptured facial expression, which reflects the effect upon mind and body of this kind of attention. Picture, for instance, the look upon the face of an enraptured lover, an entranced concertgoer, or a satisfied gourmet.[5] When a creative artist or professional athlete effortlessly performs a well-learned behavior, or a dancer becomes so absorbed in the music and her movement that she loses a sense of self, that is immersed attention. Both diffuse and immersed attention are organized by the right hemisphere of the brain.

We can pay attention in more than one way at a time. Different styles of attention are separate mechanisms and are not mutually exclusive. One can, for example, combine narrow attention with immersed, objective, or diffuse forms of attention. A fully flexible central nervous system is not biased toward the high-arousal narrow-objective focus or the low-arousal diffuse-immersed state. Instead, left to its devices, the nervous system naturally cycles through these styles, along a spectrum, and combines the variety of attention styles.

In Open Focus our attention is inclusive—sights, sounds, and other sensory information are all taken in along with space in a broadly interested way; no one sensory signal is focused on to the exclusion of the others. Most important, Open Focus allows us to be aware of how we are attending, which allows us to decide on and quickly emphasize the most appropriate styles to use. Each of the four quadrants (A, B, C, and D) defined by the intersecting lines in figure 2 corresponds to a different combination of attention styles.

Quadrant A is associated with *narrow-objective* attention, which is the style we favor most. It is an energetic and fast-paced activity that engages the brain's high frequencies (mid to high beta) and is organized primarily by the left brain. In narrow-objective focus, we preferentially attend to a limited field of experience—consisting of visual, auditory, and cognitive stimuli—while excluding internal physical sensations, emotions, and other sense modalities. This style accentuates objectification of a figure and apportions little or no awareness to the background. At its extreme it approaches one-pointed attention, for example, objectifying a candle flame.

Extreme narrow-objective attention can be crippling when it is overused or chronic, bringing on anxiety, panic, worry, and a profound generalized rigidity. It is also the enemy of a smooth, fluid performance. For example, a golfer who suffers what is known as the yips—spastic uncontrollable muscle movements when putting—is hyper-focused, and her muscles are tense.

51

Diffuse-objective attention, represented by quadrant B, occurs when we simultaneously include a wide field of experience but remain objective and separate from that experience. With this style of attention, we perceive an array of objective sensations as being suspended in the midst of a more general diffuse awareness of space, silence, mind, and timelessness. This style is typified by well-learned behaviors, over which we have gained considerable mastery through repetition. Playing in an orchestra, driving a car, performing clerical tasks, engaging in athletic or artistic performance, directing a play—all are situations in which our focus may be broadened to include a number of stimuli while we maintain a distant perspective on our performance.

Quadrants A and B both represent types of attention that depend upon remoteness from experience. The remaining two quadrants, in contrast, represent forms of attending associated with degrees of immersion in one's experience. The extreme form of immersion includes a loss of self-consciousness. While quadrants A and B emphasize the distinction and distance between self and other, subject and object, quadrants C and D emphasize dissolution of this distinction and union with experience.

The quadrant-C mode, *diffuse-immersed* attention, is an antidote to the narrow-objective style that our culture seems to demand. It is the most effective attention style in allowing us to recover from the accumulated physiological and psychological stresses wrought by modern life. Diffuse-immersed attention involves both moving into union with experience and diffusing the attentional scope of our experience at the same time. Awareness of situations that emphasize these qualities are unusual in our culture, and most often we associate this style of attention with extremes of creativity, love, and spiritual attainment. Boundaries of time and space seem to dissolve or lose definition when our attentional emphasis is on diffuse-immersed styles. While narrow-objective attention supports analysis, diffuse-immersed styles support integration of variables. Conscious awareness and flexible application of the various styles of attention lead to optimization of function.

Quadrant D represents *narrow-immersed* attention. Associated with a combination of low and high frequencies, narrow-immersed attention is a way of attending that allows us to simultaneously savor and intensify an experience. When we become absorbed in a task or lose ourselves in our work, losing a sense of time in the process, this also is narrow-immersed attention.[6] Think of a man who enjoys fishing. He forgets himself for hours as he fluidly casts his fly and sees nothing else as he waits for a fish to bite. Perhaps part of the appeal of fishing is the physiological release that comes from this style of immersed attention.

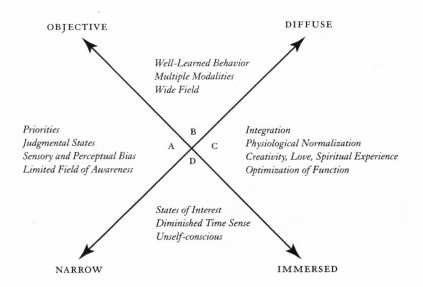

Fig. 3. The Dimensions of Attention with Associated Characteristics

Narrow-immersed attention also includes intellectually interesting or emotionally and physically pleasant and stimulating activities—any experience we want to move physically closer to in order to intensify and savor the experience. Part of the attraction of athletic or cultural events is the opportunity to become absorbed or immersed with minimum self-consciousness. And it may explain the irritation people have when they are disrupted from such deep involvement.

In addition to the composite styles of attention described by these four quadrants, we can learn to integrate the two opposing poles on either axis of attention. The importance of doing this with narrow and diffuse focus was discussed above. Maintaining objective and immersed styles of attention simultaneously is a great stress release that can change our lives. Not only do we feel more fully alive as we merge with the world, but we may find ourselves introduced to creative, transcendent realms and a multidimensional experience of life.

While all of these ways of attending are indeed part of our biological equipment, you can't just look up from this book and instantly see in Open Focus. We are too habituated to living in narrow-objective or narrow-immersed focus to break out of it that quickly. Open Focus is not just about taking in peripheral awareness but also involves rendering all objects and space with an equal and simultaneous awareness—a subtle but crucial and unmistakable difference. It is a skill that takes time and practice to learn. With some specialized exercises, however, including those in this book, anyone can learn to change the way they pay attention, and thus choose to reduce extreme attention biases and associated effort, tension, and stress accumulation.

4

What Lies Beneath: Anxiety

Anxiety is the state of
twentieth-century man.

— NORMAN MAILER,
The Naked and the Dead

TRACY, A NEW Jersey mother, was so gripped by panic attacks and agoraphobia that she was often unable to leave her home. These attacks came on suddenly, seemingly from out of nowhere, causing her heart to race, stealing her breath, and making her feel faint. She could no longer drive because the stress of being on the turnpike would sometimes trigger attacks, and she rarely left her house unless her husband drove her.

She came to see me one winter's day, started Open-Focus training in the office, and took home recorded exercises. Twice a day she listened to the exercises at home and came in to the office for biofeedback training once a week. After a few weeks her panic attacks diminished; six weeks into the training, they disappeared altogether. Tracy was elated when, on a sunny spring day, she was able to drive herself twenty-five miles to the clinic alone.

For the next twenty years she was nearly symptom free. Then, as her daughter's wedding grew near, her panic attacks returned. She nearly stopped breathing, her throat closed, she couldn't swallow even her own saliva, and she was rushed to the hospital. For days she was fed intravenously and continued to gasp for air. A week before the wedding she asked for me. I went to the hospital and coached her, in her hospital bed, in Open Focus. Her throat slowly opened and her swallowing was restored. Tracy was improved enough to attend her daughter's wedding, after which her symptoms were further alleviated.

Anxiety, from the Latin for "a lasting state of fearfulness," is the biggest mental health problem of our time. An estimated twenty million people in the United States suffer from anxiety disorders, including generalized anxiety disorder, phobias, post-traumatic stress disorder, obsessive-compulsive disorder, and panic disorder. The *Journal of Clinical Psychiatry* estimates that anxiety disorders cost the United States more than $42 billion a year—one-third of the nation's total mental-health budget. And for every diagnosed case of anxiety disorder there are many more that are not diagnosed or that occur at a level of intensity that people learn to cope with.

While anxiety is usually viewed as a mental disorder, it is really the product of our mode of living perpetually in narrow-objective attention, furthering a chronic engagement of fight or flight that has kept fearful, high-intensity memories and feelings repressed in body and mind. Faulty attention is not the only cause for the accumulation of anxiety—genetics and environment play a role; but whatever other causes there may be, attention is a fundamental and controllable factor.

A chronic emergency mode of attending doesn't always result in just classic clinical anxiety but also in a much wider range of problems. Because of genetic and environmental differences, high-frequency electrical activity in the brain manifests differently in different people. Its effects can destabilize the entire mind-body system and contribute to a host of problems, from apprehension to worry, emotional reactivity, impulsivity, and impatience.

Many cases of depression are a product of living in a chronic emergency mode of attention; a nervous system that has struggled to repress anxiety for so long becomes worn out. Quite often anxiety and depression exist simultaneously and are used to control each other. One can repress anxiety unconsciously, leaving one depressed but less anxious. Some recent research on depression supports the view that depression is caused by an overactive stress response (in other words, by chronic anxiety).[1]

In my view, narrow-objective attention contributes to the occurrence and worsening of many symptoms, from migraines to insomnia, chronic pain, stuttering, bruxism (or teeth grinding), tics, and many other problems. In my clinical experience, narrow-focus attention is also at the root of the most common disorder of attention—the inability to pay sustained interested attention in a relaxed way—which is known as attention deficit disorder or attention-deficit/hyperactivity disorder.

ANXIETY AND ADD/ADHD

Ronald, a marketing and advertising executive, didn't know he had an attention problem—a serious attention problem—until he brought his young cousin to our clinic to be treated for ADD. As his cousin was asked about some of his symptoms, Ron realized that they were similar to what he had experienced as far back as he could remember. He had never thought of them as a clinical problem but had always just thought of himself as ram-bunctious and hyper. Yet as he listened to his cousin, it dawned on him that he had suffered a serious problem all his life, some-thing now called attention-deficit/hyperactivity disorder, or ADHD. He remembered a difficult and frustrating childhood of tears and screaming, of not being able to sit still or pay atten-tion, of impulsive and often destructive behavior. "Now I know why I flunked out of three nursery schools," he said.

By current estimates, 2 to 4 percent of the adult U.S. popu-lation is affected by ADHD, causing lifelong problems for peo-ple who are otherwise often bright, energetic, and successful. Those affected by ADHD usually manage to cope with their symptoms. Indeed, after earning a degree in psychology and an MBA from the Wharton School of Business, Ron had gone on to build a successful marketing business.

After seeing positive changes in his cousin with Open-Focus training, Ron came in for his own attention training. After a single one-hour session his lifelong edginess—which he had long ago learned to live with and often didn't even real-ize he had—subsided considerably. At the end of four sessions, he felt more relaxed than he had in years, as if he had awak-ened from a long, satisfying nap. A month later, with twice-weekly clinical sessions and daily home-practice sessions, Ron found that his life was dramatically different: He was sleeping through the night and felt calm and centered. His anxiety had dissolved. Friends remarked on the change. And he had the ability to read or write for long periods of time, something that used to be difficult.

Currently attention deficits are viewed as occurring in three subtypes: predominantly inattentive (which, for the purposes of this discussion, I will simply call ADD), predominantly hyperactive/impulsive (ADHD), and combined (inattention with hyperactivity and impulsivity). All of these are, in my experience, rooted in an attention style chosen, unconsciously, to avoid underlying anxiety. Researchers have found that when children with ADHD are asked to sit quietly and look at a blank computer screen they start to feel anxious after a few minutes, as background levels of anxiety begin to surface.[2] When this happens in a classroom, as many teachers know, the ADHD student needs to start moving and doing something stimulating in order to keep from feeling the rising and powerful discomfort of anxiety. Those with ADD, on the other hand, deal with feelings of anxiety with a kind of mild dissociation: daydreaming, fantasizing, distancing themselves from the here and now. This keeps them away from the discomfort of anxiety but also prevents them from paying attention to what's in front of them.

The problem with ADD/ADHD children is not that they can't attend; it's that when they become anxious and tense they perceive this tension as boredom, which compromises their ability to attend. For these kids the greatest difficulties come at school, where they have to sit still in their seats and usually don't find the assignments engaging enough to adequately distract them from their feelings of anxiety. Put them in front of a video game, however, and they can attend for hours, because it deeply engages them and successfully distracts them from their anxiety.

Many people ask me about video games: Are they good or bad for children? Kids definitely thrive on the sense of control and mastery they get from video games. Perhaps this is a major factor leading to the addictive use and abuse of video games. Unfortunately, video games almost exclusively reward and thereby encourage narrow-objective focus, which, when overused, creates more anxiety, more overarousal, more overreactivity. Video games would be far better for the development of attention flexibility skills if they varied the styles of attention needed to perform well. For example, if knowing what was happening on the corners of the screen allowed them to score points, kids could play these games in a more relaxed, open, and even multisensory, diffuse style of attention, at least part of the time.

Why do children have such anxiety? It's a complex problem: the product of a busy and demanding world, parental and peer pressure, emotional crises that occur along a spectrum of mild to severe, and a genetic predisposition that is greater among some children than others. Some studies show that one of the most critical aspects of children's health is how secure they feel. The fear of rejection or abandonment strongly shapes a developing child's personality. Dependent on others for their survival, infants and young children are hardwired to connect to a caregiver. If that connection appears to be in jeopardy they become fearful. A climate of fear, abuse, and neglect—and, according to researchers, a lack of love and support, or even a perceived lack of love and support—engages the fight-or-flight response and prepares the child's body and mind for emergency.

"The prime directive of the brain," writes Dr. Bruce Perry, a psychiatrist who is an expert on childhood trauma and one of numerous researchers studying the fundamental role that stress plays in the human experience, "is to promote survival and procreation." He goes on:

> The brain is "overdetermined" to sense, process, store, perceive, and mobilize in response to threatening information from the external and internal environments. All areas of the brain and body are recruited and orchestrated for optimal survival tasks during the threat. This total neurobiological participation is important in understanding how a traumatic experience can impact and alter functioning in

such a pervasive fashion. Cognitive, emotional, social, be-havioral, and physiological residue of a trauma may impact an individual for years—even a lifetime.[3]

In a study conducted on the Caribbean island of Dominica, anthropologist Mark Flinn found that the relationships chil-dren have with their parents are the single biggest stress factor in their lives. Because the human brain, compared to those of other species, is still relatively unformed in childhood, human babies vitally need their parents. When children are scolded by their mothers, their level of cortisol (the stress hormone associ-ated with the fight-or-flight response) often rises by as much as 60 percent and then drops precipitously back to normal.[4] When the mother and father in one family were separated for a year, cortisol levels in their two children shot up throughout the year of the separation and then slowly dropped when the parents were reunited, though not back to normal. Higher lev-els lingered for years. Chronically high levels of cortisol cause a kind of cortisol poisoning, impairing our memory, our cogni-tive abilities, and our immune system. "There is nothing more important to a child than figuring out what makes those close to them happy and what makes them sad," Flinn says.[5] Our children are awash in anxiety-producing situations they don't understand and think they are powerless to change.

BREAKING FREE FROM CHRONIC ANXIETY AND ITS EFFECTS

The good news is that the nervous system is malleable and the chronic symptoms of increased stress can be reversed. To begin releasing long-held anxiety, we need to deemphasize narrow-objective attention and move into Open Focus, using Open-Focus exercises. When we learn to become more flexible in shifting our style of attention, we find that our physiology starts to normalize as effective training begins.

The human body comprises more than 650 separate muscles. In infants and children, muscles are exquisitely sensitive to emotions and to stress. (A number of researchers, for example, have found that the muscles of infants respond to sound, especially a mother's speech. Some research shows that a newborn responds to different phonemes in the mother's speech with the movement of different muscle groups.)[6] Indeed, humans of all ages are sensitive to stress on the muscular level. Muscles tense throughout our bodies to keep us from feeling the unpleasant stress that occurs in the emergency mode of attending. Some of those muscles can stay tensed for years or even a lifetime. It's as if the energy of fear gets trapped in the muscles. The fear is not gone, though; it's just hidden from consciousness. In addition to keeping the feeling of fear locked in our bodies, tense muscles can also cause chronic pain. To finally release our underlying anxiety, we need to dwell in Open Focus, which gradually wakes up this tension to be felt again, and then released. When we find the tension, it is a gift—for once it is made conscious, it can be completely dissolved.

If we live our lives resisting painful memories and feelings, we come to fear our present experience; and if we organize our lives to avoid discomfort, we separate ourselves from life in the moment. Or we simply focus narrowly away from the unwanted inner feelings, distancing ourselves from emotional awareness and any unpleasant manifestations in our bodies. We lose a sense of flow in our lives; we become cut off from the moment, numbed out, and separated from the intimacy of the full here-and-now experience. This kind of reality, managed around tension, is flat and dull compared to the vivid experience of life in Open Focus.

Exercise

Head and Hands
in Open Focus

THIS OPEN-FOCUS exercise is designed to begin unlocking some of the stress we carry in our head, neck, shoulders, arms, hands, and fingers. Our head and neck muscles are especially vulnerable to stress and tension because they are used prominently to support a chronic narrow-objective, gripping style of attention. This exercise is included on the audio CD that accompanies this book.

PREPARATION

Take a moment now to adjust your posture, sitting or standing, gently erect. Adopt a posture that you can maintain without the need for adjustment for the duration of the exercise. To the best of your ability, refrain from moving throughout the exercise, since this distracts one from building alternative attention styles. Can you

imagine letting your mind and body naturally and effortlessly respond to the following questions concerning
your ability to imagine certain experiences? It is usually
easier to imagine or realize the experience of space, initially emphasizing the feeling of space, with the eyes
closed.

GUIDING QUESTIONS

Can you imagine not giving any particular effort to listening to the questions or to achieving any of the associated
images or experiences? Can you imagine that the ideal response is whatever spontaneously happens to your multisensory imagery or experience when a particular question
is asked? The nature of your experience will naturally
change and deepen with continued practice. Can you
imagine that your opening and expanding awareness of
your emerging experience is a continuing process? Can
you imagine giving emphasis to imagining the feeling of
space?

Can you imagine the distance or space between your
eyes?

Is it possible for you to imagine the space inside your nose
as you inhale and exhale naturally?

Can you imagine your breath flowing behind your eyes as
you inhale naturally?

Can you imagine the distance between your nose and your eyes?

Can you imagine the space inside your throat as you inhale naturally?

Is it possible for you to imagine the space inside your throat and the space inside your nose?

Can you imagine the space inside your mouth and cheeks?

Is it possible for you to imagine the surface of your tongue?

Is it possible for you to imagine the entire region contained within your tongue—that is, can you imagine the volume of your tongue? That is, can you imagine the space your tongue occupies?

Can you imagine the space your teeth and gums occupy?

Can you imagine the volume of your lips? That is, can you imagine the space your lips occupy?

Is it possible for you to imagine the distance or space between your upper lip and the base of your nose?

Can you imagine the distance between the inside of your throat and the tip of your chin?

Can you imagine the space inside your ears?

Is it possible for you to imagine the distance between the space inside your throat and the space inside your ears?

Can you imagine the distance between the tip of your chin and the space inside your ears?

Can you imagine the space between your ears?

Can you imagine the space between the tip of your chin and your temples?

Can you imagine the distance between your temples?

Can you imagine the distance between the tip of your chin and the top of your head?

Can you imagine the space between the tip of your chin and the back of your neck?

Can you imagine the distance between the tip of your chin and your cheekbones?

Can you imagine the space between your cheekbones?

Is it possible for you to imagine the space between the tip of your chin and your eyes?

Can you imagine the space between your eyes?

Can you imagine the distance between the tip of your chin and the middle of your forehead?

Can you imagine the distance between the tip of your chin and the corners of your mouth?

Can you imagine the distance between the tip of your chin and your lower lip?

Can you imagine the distance between the corners of your mouth and your nostrils?

Is it possible for you to imagine the volume of your entire jaw?

Can you imagine the distance between your nostrils?

Can you imagine the space inside the bridge of your nose?

Can you imagine the distance between the space inside the bridge of your nose and the back of your head?

Can you imagine the distance between the space inside the bridge of your nose and your eyes?

Is it possible for you to imagine that the region around your eyes is filled with space?

Can you imagine the volume of your eyelids?

Can you imagine the distance between your eyelids and your eyebrows?

Is it possible for you to imagine the volume of your forehead?

Can you imagine the distance between the space inside the bridge of your nose and a point in the middle of your forehead?

Can you imagine the distance between the space inside the bridge of your nose and your hairline?

Is it possible for you to imagine the volume of your entire face simultaneously, including your ears, your jaw, your nose and your tongue, teeth, gums, and lips?

Can you imagine at the same time the volume of your scalp?

Can you imagine that as you inhale naturally your breath fills the entire volume of your face and scalp and head, including your ears and jaw and eyes?

Can you imagine that as you exhale and as your breath leaves your body it leaves your face, scalp, and head empty—that is, filled with space?

Can you imagine the space inside your throat expanding until your entire neck is filled with space?

Can you imagine the distance between the space inside your neck and the tips of your shoulders?

Can you imagine the space inside your throat and neck expanding to fill the entire region of your shoulders?

Can you imagine the volume of your upper arms?

Is it possible for you to imagine the volume of your upper and lower arms simultaneously?

Can you imagine the volume of your arms, wrists, and hands simultaneously?

Is it possible for you to imagine the volume of your thumbs?

Can you imagine the volume of your index fingers?

Is it possible for you to imagine the space between your thumb and index finger on each hand?

Can you imagine the volume of your middle finger on each hand?

Can you imagine the space between your index finger and your middle finger on each hand?

Can you imagine the space between your middle finger and thumb on each hand?

Is it possible for you to imagine the volume of your ring finger on each hand?

Can you imagine the space between your middle and ring fingers?

Can you imagine the space between your ring finger and thumb on each hand?

Can you imagine the volume of your little fingers?

Can you imagine the space between your ring and little fingers?

Can you imagine the space between your little finger and thumb on each hand?

Is it possible for you to imagine the volume of all of your fingers simultaneously and at the same time imagine the space between all of your fingers?

Can you imagine the volume of your shoulders, arms, hands, and fingers and at the same time imagine feeling the space between your fingers and the distance or space between your arms?

Can you imagine that as you inhale naturally your breath fills your entire head, neck, shoulders, arms, hands, and fingers and that as you exhale and as your breath leaves your body it leaves this entire region filled with space?

While remaining aware of the space inside this entire region, is it possible for you also to imagine the space around these regions—space around and between your fingers, space between your arms, space around your arms and shoulders and neck and head?

While remaining aware of the boundaries between the space inside and outside these regions, can you imagine the space freely permeating and flowing through these boundaries?

Can you imagine that as you continue to practice these Open-Focus exercises your experience will become more vivid and more effortless?

Can you imagine practicing this exercise at least twice daily?

5

Dissolving Physical Pain

ON A VISIT to an Indian reservation, a psychologist friend of mine, who is well trained in Open Focus, was invited to take part in a ceremonial sweat lodge. These lodges are small tents with hot, steaming rocks, something like a sauna. The mood among the group inside the lodge was quiet and meditative. After a few minutes the intense heat overwhelmed him. His throat and sinuses burned in pain and he fought the urge to rush out of the tent. Then his Open-Focus training came into play—he opened his attention, which drained the tension from his muscles and allowed him to merge with his discomfort; instantaneously the pain vanished. Soon, almost everyone left the tent, save the psychologist, the medicine man, and his apprentice.

After some time the medicine man reached into the pile of rocks in the center of the tent and removed a single large stone, turning it over and over in his hands, examining it slowly. Then he handed the stone—which was blistering hot—to the psychologist. His immediate reaction was to drop it, but again his Open-Focus training reflexively came into play. He stopped focusing narrowly on the hot stone, opened his awareness, and effortlessly melted into and dissolved the pain. The burning immediately stopped. Then, following the lead of the medicine man, the psychologist turned the stone over slowly in his hands to examine it before passing it to the medicine man's apprentice. The apprentice quickly put the stone down and departed.

When the two men left the sweat lodge together, the medicine man turned to the psychologist and asked, "Where did you learn to do that?"

THE TRUE SOURCE OF PAIN

Pain is epidemic in our culture. Pain is not just a throbbing headache or an aching neck but can be a broad range of sensations. I define pain as any sensation or feeling that has an unpleasant or unwanted quality or intensity of experience that lingers over time. This also includes a wide array of emotions, such as anxiety, hatred, sadness, embarrassment, loneliness, and depression. It includes all forms of physical pain—sharp, pulsating, shooting, dull, or fuzzy—even such vague forms as weltschmerz (literally "world pain"). And it includes such everyday pains as headaches, muscle spasms, back pain, and body aches.

Culturally we hold a one-dimensional view of pain, the "telegraph-wire" model. Injured tissue, this model holds, sends pain signals to our brain, where the pain is perceived. Surgeons can either cut the wire to interrupt the transmission or drug the pain into submission. Some models of pain, however, hold that tissue damage is only a small part of the total picture. A host of other physical and psychological factors determine how pain is perceived, affecting everything from the intensity of the pain to its nature, whether the pain is sharp or dull or throbbing to how other neural signals may enhance or compete with the pain. But we rarely take into account what I believe is the largest factor in the perception of pain, which is how we pay attention to it.

In simple terms, the central nervous system is responsible for perceiving and registering pain. If it is running at too high a speed and is unstable—as it is in narrow-objective attention, where we gain speed in exchange for stability—it does a poor job of handling pain signals. It becomes much more reactive and hypersensitive, registering pain that might not have any physical cause and making minor pain seem much worse than it is. Pain, then—even physical pain—is a product of how we habitually attend. Chronic narrow-objective attention, which is the style of attention that we use when we tough it out, unconsciously pushing the pain away and keeping it at bay by averting our attention, actually makes things worse.

The wide-ranging problems caused by a destabilized, over-reactive brain can be seen in the use of a drug called Neurontin, which was developed as an antiseizure medication. Seizures are the product of a brain that is electrically unstable and either can't resist, or is too easily recruited by, the spreading of certain low-frequency brain waves. Neurontin works well for seizures, and—no surprise—for a wide range of other problems, from panic attacks to migraines to eating disorders to ADD/ADHD to obsessive-compulsive disorder to chronic pain. Why? Because all of these symptoms are, in large measure, products of an electrically unstable or overactive brain. Drugs can be helpful, of course, but they have side effects, and taking a drug doesn't teach us how to establish stable brain activity or stable attention on our own.

Jack Dreyfus, the founder of the Dreyfus Fund, wrote a book called *The Story of a Remarkable Medicine*. He had suffered from serious depression for more than five years. He took the drug phenytoin (brand name Dilantin), and within an hour, he said, his symptoms went away. He talked to several others with similar stories. So impressed by his healing was Dreyfus that he launched a campaign to get the word out about the miracle of phenytoin, and now it is used around the world to treat everything from depression to anxiety, pain, mood disorders, sleep disturbances, bed-wetting, asthma, migraines, arthritis, and other problems. And just like Neurontin, Dilantin is an antiseizure medication.

A brain that can be electrically stable when necessary—and flexible when necessary—can deal with pain much more effectively than one that is not. My own clinical experience and research has shown that Open-Focus training can guide us to deploy our attention so as to achieve greater brain stability and flexibility. All pain, even the most physical (for example, from tissue damage), can be eliminated—or, at the very least, greatly mitigated—by managing the way we attend to it.

Moving Toward—Not Away— from Pain

My clinical experience shows that to effectively deal with pain we need to do the opposite of what we usually do. When we feel pain, we automatically want to distance ourselves from it and fight it, thinking that resisting or otherwise avoiding the pain will give us some relief. But over the long term exactly the reverse is true. We give power to pain by narrowly objectifying away from it, whether consciously or unconsciously. By contrast, moving toward pain in Open Focus allows it to diffuse into a broader awareness and thus to dissipate and dissolve. Clients tell me that when they bruise a knee or shin they are able to dissolve the impact quickly by using their Open-Focus skills to melt into the pain; they also report being able to reduce the symptoms of colds and speed the healing of cuts in the same

74

way. It's possible that accepting pain instead of fighting it could prevent swelling and inflammation.

The act of narrowing and objectifying attention on a painful leg, for example, holds the pain at a distance and triggers additional nervous-system arousal, which makes the brain more reactive and the leg more painful, which in turn coincides with more narrow-objective attention; as a result, the pain takes on an exaggerated place in our narrow awareness. This feedback loop tends to sustain the emergency form of attention once it is triggered, and thus it takes some time to recover electrical and attentional stability.

As a person includes diffuse attention, along with narrow focus on pain, his or her physiological arousal levels are lowered and a broadened awareness develops around the pain. Opening to and accepting pain, and moving even closer to it, in this broadened scope of attention, diminishes its intensity. When our pain becomes a small portion of our total broadened awareness it becomes more acceptable, less threatening, and can readily be merged with and dissolved altogether.

Why does how we attend affect painful muscles? In fight-or-flight mode, muscles are tense. Research has found changes in muscle cells that suggest oxygen deprivation results from tension.[1] As we open our focus, both in general and around the injured area, there is a robust physiological change. How we attend affects the brain's EEG, which in turn releases muscle tension, increases blood flow, and changes a host of other functions associated with sympathetic autonomic nervous system activity and increase of parasympathetic activity.

It's easy to understand the need to alter and broaden the way we attend to the external world but harder perhaps to understand the concept of paying attention differently to internal feelings and sensations, because our reactions to these are often unconscious and automatic. But if we get caught in an inward narrow focus, it has profound effects on our day-to-day lives.

Most people are familiar with the placebo effect, the phenomenon of an ailing patient getting better when taking a fake, or "dummy," pill that he or she believes is real. The placebo effect may in fact be a result of unconsciously changing how we attend to our internal experiences. It's a powerful phenomenon: In many double-blind studies of antidepressants and other psychoactive drugs, the placebo group fares as well as or better than the group taking the actual medication. This demonstrates the powerful self-healing mechanisms we have, and this effect is usually ascribed to a patient's expectation or belief that he or she will get better.

There's no consensus on what the physiological mechanism underlying the placebo effect is, but a good case can be made that it is mediated by a shift in attention. When patients are given a placebo (a sugar pill, for example) they release their lock on a narrow-objective attention to their symptoms and include a more diffuse-immersed form of attention as they begin to merge with signs of illness, allowing symptoms to dissolve and supporting improved health.

Narrow focus on pain is like standing next to a brick wall and attending exclusively to a single brick. That's all you see and think about. It occupies all of your awareness. Make your attention more diffuse and the brick becomes one in a wall of many. Diffuse your attention a little more and the brick becomes part of a home. Diffuse even further and the brick becomes part of a neighborhood. Further still the brick becomes part of a city; yet further, part of a state and part of a country; then a continent; then the Earth, and then a part of our solar system, and so forth. This visual exercise is a form of Open-Focus training. When we allow our perception of the brick to merge with each of the above juxtapositions in turn, and then all at once, the perception of the brick diffuses, dissipates, and dissolves in every direction and through peripheral awareness.

THE PROCESS OF PAIN REDUCTION

The process of dissolving pain begins by establishing a physically quiet, low-frequency style of attention. Some trainees can move quickly toward Open Focus, while others may need more time and may need to practice with a recorded exercise. Once clients in diffuse attention have objectified their pain and the space in, around, and through it, they imagine moving toward the pain, eventually merging with it. Others may prefer allowing the pain to wash over them until they are bathing in it. In either case, the pain is no longer held exclusively as an object at a distance in narrow focus; we have now diffused our awareness around it and merged with it and let it wash through our diffuse awareness of pain, and let it spread further.

It's also possible to learn to imagine narrowing focus on the precise location of pain and consciously diving into the heart of it, as I did with kidney-stone pain. It's like knowing the water is cold but you dive into a swimming pool anyway. It's a faster approach, but not everyone can do it. Some clients need to take more time to move their awareness toward the pain's physical location and its inevitable dissolution. Still others prefer to passively allow the pain to come to their location, the physical place where they locate their seat of consciousness.

To summarize the sequence of attention styles usually necessary for pain dissolution, it usually begins with the client in narrow-objective attention and at least somewhat averse to full and direct experience of the pain. The client is first guided to include in his peripheral awareness a diffuse attention to all available senses in space. This is developed while attention is centered in feeling his pain and feeling the space that pervades all sensations. Keeping this diffuse attention in awareness, the second step is to narrow and objectify the pain by physically feeling its location in the body, feeling its shape, and feeling its intensity (on a zero-to-ten scale). The third step establishes a clearer, more direct objective attention to the pain with a simultaneous diffuse experience of space and sensations as a background. The fourth attention change involves creating the permissive conditions for merging one's conscious awareness into the center or heart of the experience of pain, thus allowing it to spread, diffuse, dissipate, and dissolve over a period of one to thirty seconds.

A number of repetitions of this sequence may be necessary to completely dissolve the pain. Complete rather than partial dissolution of pain makes it less likely that that pain will return after the exercise is ended. Resumption of pain is directly related to how quickly the person returns to the conditioned or biased forms of attention they are accustomed to. Maintenance of Open Focus, a roughly equal presence of the four styles of attention, is the long-term goal, a balanced state that is the preferred solution for a host of stress-related symptoms. These attention changes can be effective in one or a few sessions for emotional and even physical tissue damage related to pain. However, it is recommended that medical and psychological professionals be consulted to rule out underlying, untoward, serious, life-threatening conditions associated with chronic and recurrent pain and toxic emotion.

Repression and chronic avoidance of pain causes an immense energy drain, and once pain has been dissolved it frees up energy for other things. Clients who have dissolved their pain—physical and emotional—using Open-Focus skills often feel more centered, as if they have slipped back into their own "skin" after a long absence.

6

Dissolving
Emotional Pain

GEORGIA HAD suffered anxiety at low levels for many years. Like many clients, she learned how subconsciously to suppress the anxiety that rose in her, and how to use her anxiety to lift her up when she felt depressed. Like many she also managed her anxiety by distracting herself with activities such as watching movies, shopping, or working out at the gym, in addition to working long hours.

As she grew older, however, stress accumulated and the distraction strategy Georgia had used no longer served her. Perhaps the most pressing problem arose out of her worrying about the health of an aged parent she cared for. Between elder care, her demanding job as a civil servant, and her own health needs over a period of years, she began to feel emotionally overwhelmed. The stress-induced anxiety she had accumulated earlier in her life compounded her current stress. Other symptoms, including insomnia, grief, loneliness, a feeling of isolation, and physical pain had also emerged—a common phenomenon when repression of anxiety is prolonged.

Georgia came to see me and described her symptoms. She didn't know that all her symptoms were connected; she only came in to deal with her anxiety. She felt she was losing control because when a generalized feeling of anxiousness came it would last at high levels for days, and there was nothing she could do for it. She occasionally took Xanax, but it made her tired and she worried about forming a dependency.

She started working with brain synchrony and Open-Focus training after her intake session. The goal was to allow her physiology to quiet to the point that she could feel the source of her anxiety as a physical event. While the source of physical pain is usually easy to find, emotional pain can be more difficult to localize, even though noxious emotions usually have a source in the body. If we can sit still and access the brain's lower frequencies, we can easily be taught to open up to the source of these painful feelings in the body. Common places for emotions are in the stomach, the neck, or the chest, or a whole-body generalized feeling of anxiety; but emotional pain can reside anywhere in the body. When feelings or emotions—or physical pain sometimes—are not immediately experienced as localized events in the body, then a series of guiding questions can lead attention to an awareness of the bodily locations of the strongest feelings. Finding the site or source of these feelings is an important step to their rapid dissolution.

Georgia had three weekly training sessions and practice at home each day to increase her brain synchrony, which increased her diffuse and immersed attention. Experiencing localized feelings, emotions, and pain within the context of this broad and immersed attention allows us to feel pain as a relatively small, low-intensity event, which prevents overreaction.

As she experienced Open Focus she was able to use the guiding questions to find, diffuse, and dissolve completely the emotions of anxiety and depression and an underlying feeling of grief. She was surprised at how quickly her anxiety responded to home practice and synchrony training during her weekly visits. At first, after a practice session, her mind was free of noxious emotion and the body feelings of anxiety for a period of hours after she dissolved it. This pain-free period was extended with continued practice. The difficulties of caring for an aged parent became less stressful and her worry about her parent's condition became more manageable. It was as if she could put down her troubles and worries for a period of time as necessary, and then pick them up when that was appropriate.

There is a general belief that emotional pain is not physical, or does not cause physical pain. Emotional pain, however, is often presented as intensely physical and, in fact, some of the most difficult pain in our lives is caused by, or exacerbated by, emotional pain, even though many physicians and mental health providers don't see it that way. They hold that pain crops up because the body is malfunctioning for some reason instead of being seen as the result of a control strategy involving efforts to mask emotion.

Take the case of a psychotherapist and her patient, who sat together quietly, listening to Open-Focus exercises, when the therapist began to feel nauseated. The next time she listened to the exercises, the nausea rose up again. The therapist soon connected this experience with memories of an eating disorder she suffered from as a teenager. Though she thought those troubles were long behind her, doing the Open-Focus exercises helped her to realize that the emotional issues surrounding her eating disorder had never been fully resolved. Instead she had simply blocked and suppressed them. Open-Focus training put her in touch with long-standing feelings of anxiety that felt rooted in her stomach, allowing her the opportunity to acknowledge and dissolve these painful feelings.

The stomach and intestines are extraordinarily sensitive to emotional stress and are places where we commonly feel anxiety and commonly block it. I believe emotional and other forms of stress are a major source of the many intestinal ailments in our culture, from common digestive disorders to irritable-bowel syndrome, and many other problems. Some researchers believe the gut possesses something like a second brain, calling it the "enteric nervous system." This nervous system is composed of a network of 500 million neurons, neurotransmitters, and proteins found in the esophagus, stomach, small intestine, and colon. It is the only large number of neurons outside the central nervous system, considered to function as a single entity, and it has cells like those in the brain and a complex circuitry that allows it to act independently, and to learn, remember, and produce what we call "gut feelings."[1]

Listening to Open-Focus exercises can awaken repressed feelings, but it normally does so in a mild and gentle way that people feel they can handle. In the case of this therapist, feelings in her stomach led her to gradually feeling and remembering past pain and anxiety. To address the uncomfortable physical sensations that came up, she used the exercise for dissolving pain (see pages 112–15). This allowed her to center her attention specifically on her stomach pain and change the way she paid attention to it, shifting from narrow-objective focus (which she had used to keep her pain at a distance for years) to Open Focus, in which she moved toward her pain and fully accepted it. As with physical pain, when emotional pain becomes part of the larger awareness of Open Focus, it's much easier to accept and diffuse. By simply learning to shift our attention, we can melt into our physical or emotional pain and dissolve it.

As Open-Focus training continues, deeper, often unacknowledged physical and emotional issues that have been long repressed can surface into conscious awareness. Because Open-Focus attention promotes a physiologically neutral and broadly inclusive state, feelings and emotions usually surface gently.

More intense "release phenomena" do occasionally occur and can be both pleasant and disturbing. These can come in the form of tingling sensations, muscle tremors, pains, aches, perspiration, and spontaneous feelings that seem to have no specific source, like waves of pleasure or emotionally charged memories. These feelings, emotions, and sensations appear to be the result of the body partially letting go of tension and repressed pain. Open-Focus attention strategies are ideally suited to dissolve these release phenomena as they arise.

WORKING WITH DEPRESSION

Tony had already been experiencing depression and anxiety when he was involved in a serious automobile accident. A truck snagged low-hanging power wires, which pulled down a telephone pole, which snapped and then fell on Tony's car and across his back. The truck that caused the accident sped away, leaving him pinned in his car by the telephone pole until he was found by another driver. Both the fact of the accident and the ongoing physical pain that it brought into Tony's life intensified a downward emotional spiral; he was in great despair about his bad luck, which in turn aggravated his tension and anxiety. He was lethargic and unhappy and would lie around his house, unable to motivate himself to get up and do anything. He tried several antidepressants, but they didn't help. His psychologist referred him for biofeedback.

In cases like Tony's, with several presenting symptoms, Open-Focus exercises are applied to the strongest sensations first. When the strongest sensations dissolve completely they also dissolve the lesser sensations of the same kind. If anxiety, for example, is the most intense feeling, I ask the client to use the Open-Focus exercise to locate this feeling in the body, to feel its shape, to rate its intensity on a one-to-ten scale, and then proceed to dissolve it with Open-Focus attention techniques. As a client dissolves high-intensity anxieties, lesser anxieties also release. And, not infrequently, unpleasant feelings that don't seem associated with anxiety also disappear.

As in Tony's case, depression is very often accompanied by anxiety and tension. I usually begin treatment for depression by dissolving the anxiety first, when the latter is present. In my view, anxiety and depression can be and often are part of the same complex problem. Most of the depression I treat is the result of an unconscious attempt to control and reduce feelings of anxiety by reflexively denying or avoiding feeling in the body. When the anxiety is dissolved the need to control anxiety by depressing oneself also disappears and depression can lift on its own or can be easily dissolved using Open-Focus exercises. In any case, resistance to feelings of depression can be dissolved directly along with the feeling of depression itself.

After three general Open-Focus training sessions Tony was introduced to the dissolving-pain exercise to start reducing his anxiety. During the first session he reported that he was only able to reduce his feelings of anxiety by about 15 percent, which is a poor result, and almost all of this anxiety returned shortly after the session. It wasn't until the sixth session that Tony was able to dissolve significant amounts of anxiety and physical pain at home and during our office sessions. I ask my clients to think about what number on a scale of zero to ten they would use to describe the intensity of their pain. During the sixth session Tony dissolved chronic spine pain from six to zero on a ten-point scale, and chronic pain in his right shoulder from four to zero. By the next session he said he was starting to feel "happy," and this was even before we started dissolving feelings of depression and sadness. By the ninth session—after we had spent two sessions dissolving feelings of depression—he said he felt 100 percent better. He continued to dissolve feelings of depression and sadness, and these were reduced to zero. His life returned to near normal, and during the tenth session he reported doing chores around his house, which he had not been able to perform since the accident.

Much of Tony's physical pain and other symptoms resulting from the accident ameliorated during the weeks that we focused on his anxiety and depression. Tony's case illustrates the way in which narrow-objective focus upon pain greatly exacerbates the experience of pain and how changing to diffuse-immersed attention eases even extreme pain. Tony began treatment with a plethora of symptoms—pain in his spine and shoulder blades, a sense of overall heaviness and brokenness, neck and head tension, numbness, burning in his upper spine, fear in his heart, anger at the truck driver who left the scene, nightmares, waking insomnia (awaking during the night and not being able to fall back to sleep), and other negative emotions. All of these were mitigated or resolved by daily home practice of dissolving-pain techniques and office sessions of EEG-synchrony training.

It's easier to treat depression if there is anxiety (anxiety is easier to dissolve), but Open-Focus exercises can work directly by using feelings of depression, sadness, loneliness, or despair as the pain that we dissolve, instead of anxiety.

The symptoms of depression and anxiety can return, depending on how well the client learns to move—and stay—out of chronic effortful forms of narrow-objective attention and to cultivate a stable Open-Focus attention. This, in turn, is related to how often and how well they do their Open-Focus exercises and how well they can maintain Open Focus in daily life. Depression and anxiety take years to form, in both the brain and body, and they may have their roots both in genetic predisposition and in powerful situational influences in early life and beyond. When clients habitually return to a chronic narrow focus they bring on these feelings again. Thus, I encourage people to use these negative feelings as feedback. If they start to feel anxious or depressed, or if other unpleasant feelings return, these experiences can serve as a reminder to move back into Open Focus, which allows stress, tension, and other unwanted feelings to dissipate. The pain becomes feedback. At some point clients are sufficiently better that they can reduce coming for treatment. We instruct clients to continue to dissolve layers of repressed emotion until they can welcome the process of being open to feelings, and have the confidence to dissolve them by themselves at home.

WORKING WITH TRAUMA, POST-TRAUMATIC STRESS DISORDER (PTSD)

At the Vietnam Veterans Memorial in Washington, D.C., a combat veteran named Rob was showing his daughter the names of people who had served alongside him. During his tour of duty, Rob had seen several men get killed and had also witnessed other tragic events.

That day, a young, active-duty soldier who was also visiting the wall overheard Rob talking to his daughter and asked him if he had served. Rob said he had, and the soldier extended his hand to Rob and said, "Welcome home, sir." Out of nowhere, Rob broke into great heaving sobs. He had to be held to keep from falling down on the spot. It took an hour before he was able to walk away. He had buried the intensity of his trauma for many years, in body and mind, remaining unconscious of it until that moment.

This story suggests how long we can carry and how deeply we can repress traumatic memories. Open-Focus training can help us become aware of these kinds of repressed feelings and dissolve them as they arise. You might be thinking, "Why would I want to dredge up these kinds of long-buried feelings? Isn't that asking for trouble?" But even though these problems are buried, the negative feelings are not lost and the tension and energy necessary to repress any highly charged experience takes a tremendous toll on us physically and psychologically. Repressed trauma affects nearly every aspect of our lives. As these tensions and emotions surface and dissolve in Open Focus, life changes for the better.

At the same time, it is not unusual in our clinic to dissolve the residual emotions and tensions of a long-forgotten trauma without the patient remembering or reliving the situation of the traumatizing event itself. The event may later be remembered without much or any attendant emotion or tension. This may occur when the emotional pain is clearly localized in the body, and is not just a mental event, that is, "only in one's mind."

STRESS AND VISION

One body region where we accumulate a great deal of pain and tension, both emotional and physical, is our eyes. At one level, the eye is changed by physical stress because of how we use it. From an evolutionary perspective, humans paid attention very differently for most of their history than they do now. In the days of hunters and gatherers, people varied their attention— looking at expansive views and scanning the horizon for the movement of game part of the time. Focusing narrowly as they carved a tool or painted a picture was just a small part of how they paid attention. Now narrow-objective focus dominates our day. Sitting in front of a computer or performing a repetitive task on a factory assembly line for hours and days on end can cause serious eye strain. Forcing ourselves to pay extra, sustained attention to things we need—rather than desire—to see causes even more eyestrain, which in turn leads to everything from headaches to neck and shoulder pain. In his book *The Art of Seeing,* Aldous Huxley wrote: "A small boy studying algebra exhibits voluntary attention—that is if he exhibits any attention at all. The same boy playing a game exhibits spontaneous attention. Voluntary attention is always associated with effort and tends more or less rapidly to produce fatigue."

Emotional stress may have an even greater impact on our eyes than physical stress. Because they are so vital to making our way in the world, responding to fear and being vigilant to assure our safety, the muscles of the eye are among the most sensitive to emotional stress. (Remember Kyle, the boy from chapter 1 who grew up in a threatening environment and had trouble reading?) Growing up, all of us at times feel unsafe and threatened in our environment, which leads to chronic narrow focus and to tension of the eye and face muscles. This distorts the eyeball, restricts its movement, and affects vision. We can learn to gain some control over our eye muscles and release the tension and pain we carry in them. Doing so is advisable because these muscles are often fixated and warped out of their healthy state by a lifetime of chronic stress. Indeed, a small number of researchers have long maintained that releasing tension in the eyes can greatly improve our vision.[1]

The selection and control of images falling on the eye are carried out by three delicate and distinct muscle systems, one on the outside of the eyeball and the other two inside the eye. The iris is an inner muscle that regulates the amount of light entering the eye by varying pupil diameter. Another internal muscle system is the ciliary body, a ring of muscle around the lens that adjusts the shape of the lens to bring near and far objects into focus. The third set of muscles, attached to the sclera (the outer covering of the eye), are responsible for tracking and pulling the eye in various directions to scan and search.

A number of clients who have used Open-Focus exercises that ask them to imagine space in and around their eyes report improvement of nearsightedness and other longtime vision problems; the changes are sometimes dramatic (for example, from 20/200 to 20/40) and are assumed to result from the release of tension in the muscles that control focusing and tracking. Releasing muscles of the forehead, neck, and face—all of which help support narrow focus—also helps.

Our eyes also contribute to problems with vertigo and dizziness. Jim was a client who suffered chronic dizziness and blurred vision. After a couple of sessions of Open Focus, he noticed feelings of tension at the back of his eyes. During the next session he moved toward those feelings and was able to dissolve them, bringing both his blurred vision and dizziness to an end.

STRESS AND DISEASE

Stress plays a large role in the suppression of the immune system.[2] Because the immune system defends us against so many disparate problems, the health consequences are far-reaching when it becomes compromised by stress. On the other hand, reducing the stress load with attention training can improve the immune system and dissolve a wide array of symptoms.

Kent came to see me for stress-related pain symptoms. He also suffered from chronic and severe food allergies, allergies so strong he needed daily antihistamine injections to avoid vomiting everything he ate. He could eat only a few bland foods, such as free-range chicken and organically grown brown rice and spinach, which he often threw up as well.

In addition to his phsyiological symptoms he had a difficult emotional history. His mother died when he was young, he said, and his father was distant and demanding. He was working full time as a financial consultant and was going to night school. He complained about being a perfectionist in everything he did and he felt overwhelmed with anger and exhaustion.

Although Kent felt that his pain and allergies were separate from his stress and didn't expect his work with me to help them, his food reactions seemed less severe after a brief course of attention training. He signed up for an intensive weeklong attention-training seminar. During the process he noticed feelings of fear and anger rise up, and he learned to dissolve them. Feeling good two days into the seminar, Kent decided— against my advice—to skip his usual medication and injections during the remaining program. By the end of the week he felt as good without the allergy shots as he had felt while taking them. In addition, he found that he could eat a much wider range of foods without vomiting than he could before the seminar. After a few more weeks of home training he could eat almost anything he chose.

Kent had been tested for allergies before he began Open-Focus training, and after the training he was tested again. Instead of testing negative for the long list of food allergies, he still—to my surprise—tested positive for all of the same foods as before; some tested even worse. What had changed was his body's overreaction to the allergens. (We generally ask new clients not to discontinue medications that are working without significant side effects. For many of these clients progress is slower than for those who are nonmedicated, and they make fewer gains. However, Open Focus often allows reduction or stopping of medications.)

Stabilizing the brain through Open-Focus training, and dissolving anxiety, can help people manage such problems as obsessive-compulsive disorder, stuttering, tics, Tourette's syndrome, and other problems in which the body's reactivity seems to take on a life of its own. They are all problems in which anxiety plays a large role.

One client was a young man who suffered a range of tics—head jerks, arching back, involuntary jumping, constant blinking, and some vocal noises. Most people with tic disorders find that stress exacerbates their problem and that their embarrassment over having tics in front of others causes feelings of anxiety, which in turn makes their tics worse. He went through a series of doctors and medications, finally finding one, risperidone (the brand name is Risperdal), that diminished his tics somewhat but not nearly enough for him to have the kind of life he wanted.

"When I started Open-Focus training I felt a difference right away," he wrote me. "I had a steady period of feeling good, about two weeks. Since I was feeling a lot better I started going to school and was enjoying my life better than I did in a long time." He learned how to dissolve anxiety as it rose in him whenever the tics started. "All of my tics improved, even though a few of them are still there they are not as severe as they used to be (90 percent less). Even though I don't feel 100 percent better my life has become more enjoyable."

Emotional and physical pain are equally amenable to treatment with Open-Focus training, and the following exercise can be used to treat either.

Exercise

Dissolving Pain

INTRODUCTION

ONCE YOU have learned to move into Open-Focus awareness, it becomes possible to use your attention to dissolve physical and emotional pain. In Open Focus your pain is a much smaller part of your total awareness; it becomes no big deal and is easy to accept and therefore easy to dissolve. This exercise teaches you how to move closer to pain in a broadened awareness until the pain diffuses and disappears. Simply accepting the feeling of pain while resting in Open Focus is often enough to dissolve the pain.

PREPARATION

Sit quietly, accepting potential distractions. If you have pain—a headache or muscle tension or anxiety—allow yourself to become aware of its location in your body and then feel into the pain as openly and directly as you can, without resisting it. Dissolving pain can be accomplished only after you have precisely located the feeling in your body.

1. THE SENSE INVENTORY

Gently do a mental inventory of the perceptions of all your senses. Attend, for example, to your sense of hearing. Be aware of sounds while equally and simultaneously attending to the silence between the sounds, out of which the sounds arise. Notice the direction that sounds travel toward you through three-dimensional space. Let this awareness deepen for a few seconds.

Now add vision, noticing the space and objects that you are seeing or visualizing (if your eyes are closed).

Be aware of any tastes, including the taste of space. Let this experience deepen for a few seconds.

Add an awareness of the sense of smell and even the smell of space. Sit with this experience for fifteen seconds or so.

Add an awareness of your thoughts and the mental silence from which they emerge, the silence in which they exist, and the silence into which they dissolve.

Now add an awareness of a sense of nowness, the feeling that you are in the present, experiencing all of your senses existing in present space, silence, and timelessness simultaneously.

In the center of this diffuse attention is the sense of feeling, which includes the felt presence of your body, the feeling of absence we call space around the body, and the space your body occupies. The more we increase the sense of the simultaneous presence of all our senses in space, centered in feeling, the more we deepen diffuse attention and the Open-Focus experience.

2. EXPANDING AND DISSOLVING THE PAIN

Can you imagine centering this expanded awareness on your pain? Now can you imagine feeling the space around the pain and feeling the space the pain occupies, while remaining in a diffuse peripheral awareness of available, different sense objects, and the space in which they exist?

Now allow your awareness to diffuse through the pain, feeling the pain more. Alternatively, let the pain diffuse through your awareness. Bathe in the pain. Let the pain diffuse by feeling it more—not less. Let pain spread through surrounding areas of the body and into space. Don't try to make the pain spread. It will naturally diffuse as your acceptance of feeling it is more pervasive.

You've increased the breadth of your awareness and allowed the pain to become a small part of the totality of that expanded awareness. The pain no longer encompasses all of your awareness—it's a small part and it's no big deal. Expanding your focus allows you to be more comfortable with moving into your pain, to feel the pain more. Understandably, most people try to avoid their pain. Yet what actually makes the pain overwhelming is our narrow focus on it, which allows the pain to dominate our awareness. When we open up our awareness, our pain becomes a small part of the totality of our experience and feels less threatening. It's no longer scary to merge with it and let it diffuse into surrounding body and space.

The goal of this exercise is to open our awareness and dive into and through the center of the pain and then let the awareness of pain float in an open and inclusive awareness where it can dissolve. If the pain doesn't completely and immediately dissolve, dive back into its core. Some people can dissolve their pain in one or two passes, while others require more.

We can also dissolve our pain as we carry out daily activities by maintaining a feeling sense of space and other sensations in and around our pain as we talk on the phone, shop for groceries, prepare meals, and so forth. We don't recommend—in fact, we caution against—practicing Open-Focus and dissolving-pain exercises while operating any vehicle or in potentially harmful conditions.

7

Love Is a Way of Paying Attention

Open-Focus Tools for Relationships

Dear Dr. Fehmi,
How can I relate what happened? After working with
you for some time . . . suddenly my whole being was
flooded with love. It was so powerful that I had to lie
down in the woods behind your office looking up into
the sky through the trees for a long, long time—just
filled with total unconditional love—loving the whole
universe and everyone and everything in it. A cosmic
orgasm. A major peak experience. Did this happen
because all my brain waves were in synch? You will
have to explain it scientifically. This was a big, unfor-
gettable experience that I'm very grateful to you for.
Sincerely,
Louisa

Martin was a middle manager who oversaw a dozen lower-level managers at a stock-and-bond brokerage in New York City. While he enjoyed his work and was successful, life at home was a different story. Martin was dissatisfied with his family and chronically irritable when he was with his wife and kids. He overreacted to many small details of home life, and he was aware of it, but he simply couldn't control himself. If one of the kids slammed the door or used one of his tools and didn't put it back, Martin would get angry, much angrier than the situation called for. He also suffered chronic back pain, hypertension, and headaches, and these problems seemed worse at home. He was so unhappy with his domestic life that he dreaded leaving the office for home each day and worked longer hours than his job required. He obsessively thought about divorcing his wife and leaving his family.

One day, at his wife's urging, Martin showed up for neurofeedback and Open-Focus training. After the first training session he noticed a slight positive change in his attitude, and felt a little less irritable. After a few weeks of home training and several more neurofeedback and Open-Focus sessions, Martin started to notice fundamental changes in his life. His emotional reactivity was greatly reduced. He felt significantly less irritable, his anxiety diminished, and his rages stopped. "The rough edges were smoothed," he says. He began to feel warmer and more personable, more relaxed and open, both in the office and at home.

He now paid attention to how he was attending and found he could apply flexible-attention skills while driving, reading, or even talking. If he was talking to a colleague, for example, he would relax his attention and converse in a more casual way. If he noticed the price of a stock was dropping and felt he needed to pay attention to it, he narrowed his focus but would diffuse it again as soon as he had finished. And, if he chose to, he could work longer hours without feeling drained and on edge at the end of the day.

Most important, he found himself wanting to be with his family. Relationships at home became warmer, and chronic negative thoughts dropped away. Things his wife and kids did didn't bother him that much anymore. He gave up notions of divorce. For the first time in years, Martin could cope without denying, escaping, or withdrawing, but simply by managing the style of his attention. And he came to realize that most of the problems at home resulted from how he reacted to his wife and children rather than from something they did. Living constantly in the stressful emergency mode of narrow-objective focus had made him chronically overreact to everything, but was particularly damaging to those relationships he cared about most. Even love depends on how we pay attention.

ATTENTION HABITS FORM EARLY

Our patterns of experiential avoidance are laid down early in life, based on genetics and environmental conditioning. Just as infants and toddlers exploring the world learn to avoid a hot stove or sharp objects, we learn later in childhood to avoid painful emotional experience by deploying a narrow-objective style of attention. Unfortunately, narrow-objective attention is an emergency mode that magnifies our perception of pain, which we then attempt to tamp down by reflexively tensing our muscles and turning our narrow beam of attention away from the pain.

Time passes, the painful memories accumulate, and we become addicted to narrow-objective focus, through which we can seemingly avert and distance ourselves from pain. It seems to be the only way to keep noxious experience from surfacing.

But because the tension of narrow-objective focus is chronic and general, we not only avoid—temporarily—unpleasant experiences but, in the process, also prevent pleasant ones as well. Chronic use of a narrow-objective beam of awareness divorces us from experience by separating us from the world, instead of allowing us to merge with it. We perceive rigid boundaries between ourselves and everything else, between our heart and our controlling mind. Carrying stress and past emotional wounds in our mind and body warps our perceptions; we see the world "through a glass, darkly," making the world seem more fearsome and unfriendly than it is. We feel like victims. We make poor decisions on every level. Jealousy, anger, hate, mistrust, fear, loneliness, and paranoia are largely the result of the emotional baggage we carry. This paradox is at the heart of our attention processes: by seeking to avoid these unpleasant feelings we exacerbate them.

We live in our mind, inside our heads, attending narrowly almost exclusively to thinking, seeing, and hearing, at the expense of feeling. Intellectual understanding is a pale replica of reality. The real action lies in fully experiencing love and the other pleasures being human has to offer. We crave union. We long for deep relationships with other people and the world around us.

If we wish to move toward experiences of deeper and more satisfying union, we need to tone down the exclusionary forms of attention and enhance the inclusionary and unifying forms. Love is about opening our attention and losing ourselves in our experience. Open-Focus training is about releasing, expressing, giving, accepting, and engaging in union. Sound familiar? Our quest is to promote greater brain-wave synchrony, which corresponds with opening and merging self with other. Diffuse-immersed styles of attention can dissolve the separateness, loneliness, and isolation that result from overuse of narrow-objective attention. Attention biases and attentional rigidity are the principal causes of human misery and suffering.

Love wakes up the right side of our brain and allows it to share center stage with the usually dominant left hemisphere, bringing the emotional, empathetic, and spiritual side of our nature online. This side of ourselves is evident—specifically as compassion—when we are empathic and deeply understand someone else's heartache or joy because we resonate with what it feels like, because we are on the same wavelength. Open-Focus training helps to realize love and compassion.

ATTENTION AND MARRIAGE

Margaret came to see me seeking treatment for her migraines, not her relationship. But she talked about some of the problems at home. James wanted to get married, but Margaret was too upset with his sloppiness and the disregard for her that she thought it implied. She was unwilling to commit. James felt rejected and nagged, so he turned a deaf ear to her complaints. Each nursed their grievances in narrow focus, ruminating endlessly about them. They were drifting apart and on the brink of ending their relationship. "But," Margaret said after she described her relationship, "I'm here for my migraines."

Within a very few sessions of Open-Focus training, Margaret's headaches diminished and were almost eliminated. I remember the day she came in and told me how thrilled she was to be free from pain. And then, to her surprise, she went on to describe a very different relationship with her boyfriend since doing the training. She spoke of feeling closer emotionally to him and more at ease with her life and the world. James's sloppiness was no longer a big deal, and the dirty clothes on the floor and newspapers on the couch no longer bothered her much. She became less vocal, he felt less nagged, and his messiness decreased greatly. As he improved, she felt more appreciated and became more affectionate. In short, they had "connected" again, which increased James's desire to make Margaret happy.

Happy endings like this are a potent reminder that the first order of business in healing interpersonal relationships is to teach each person in the relationship to pay attention in a way that increases acceptance and decreases his or her own emotional reactivity. Open-Focus training reduces the emotional reactivity of both parties.

The notion of people who are emotionally linked being on the same "wavelength" seems to be a real phenomenon. As part of an experiment, I wired a couple to the same biofeedback equipment but placed them in separate rooms. They only received the feedback tone and light when both were producing synchronous alpha waves within *and* between themselves. For half an hour they learned to make the feedback happen. After the training session ended they reported a "honeymoon response," an unusually close bond, leaving them feeling emotionally closer than they had for a long time. We now use this approach with other kinds of pairs—parent and child, coach and player, teammates, teacher and student, and so on. A psychologist-lawyer in Dallas, Texas, Dr. Robert Gordon, uses synchrony training with opposing parties in litigation to help them achieve conflict resolution. Similar results are possible without neurofeedback instruments by doing Open-Focus exercises together.

Marriage Therapy in Open Focus

As with other kinds of marriage counseling, Open-Focus couples therapy begins with both parties listing their symptoms and articulating their grievances. Having lost the ability to put themselves in each other's shoes, both partners in a troubled relationship feel unheard, defensive, and distant. It becomes the therapist's job to help the partners want to communicate, so that empathy can replace separateness.

In traditional couples therapy, maladaptive patterns are identified; then, through insight and shared expression, better communication skills are established, free of past conflict and pain. The Princeton Biofeedback clinic staff do the same thing, but we teach Open-Focus skills first. As Margaret's case demonstrates, grievances between two people often fall away after one or both people have stabilized their physiology with Open-Focus exercises; neurofeedback training for synchrony is optional, though ideally it is an effective contribution to the process. As a troubled relationship becomes more stressed, each person becomes increasingly preoccupied with their own pain and stuck in narrow-objective focus, which in turn makes them hypersensitive and prone to overreact. They become unwilling or unable to reach out to the other for consolation, to see the other's point of view, to behave fairly or with care, or to identify with the other person. But when both partners learn the fundamental skills of letting go and of diffusing and merging attention, they find that compassion and reconnection arise naturally. Open-Focus and synchrony training speed, guide, and enhance this process.

Couples are also asked to discuss their differences while in Open Focus. In this relaxed attention, it becomes possible for them to listen more empathetically and with less reactivity. When they get stuck or intensity levels start to rise, physical and emotional pain is diffused with dissolving-pain techniques. Often things are said in couples therapy that are hurtful; and whether or not it is necessary for these things to be said, the pain often causes couples to shut down communication.

Open Focus helps to keep communication open and enables couples to speak the truth, because they know each partner can dissolve any pain that interferes with his or her ability and willingness to listen, understand, and deeply accept the other.

CAN YOU IMAGINE?

Changing the way we attend changes much more than our relationships with other people—it changes the way we perceive and inhabit our inner and outer worlds.

In her elegant book *Sight and Sensibility: The Ecopsychology of Perception*, Laura Sewall, PhD, of Prescott University in Arizona, an expert in the psychology and neurophysiology of vision, wrote of her vision problem and the changes she experienced by practicing vision-therapy exercises. As her nearsightedness improved, she found that landscapes became more distinct and vibrant and her relationship to the world was enhanced. She writes:

> After a month or so I suddenly glimpsed sharp, razorlike edges and neon colors. . . . As I became more practiced, as I developed a kind of crafted nonchalance about this great new beckoning of the world, glimpses became long moments of rich perception.
>
> My imagination became strong and clear and I was able to picture whatever I wanted to see. The world began to light up with a newfound resonance and my resistance to the urban landscape, to Los Angeles, and to the world in general, diminished. I became more receptive to seeing the whole of what lay before my eyes. . . . Fear slipped into a previous life. . . . I was falling in love with the world and desperately curious about how my vision was stirring up such a potent mix of sensations and emotions within me.

103

The experience so astonished Sewall that she went back to school—earning a doctorate in neuropsychology—in order to understand what was happening to her. People who practice Open Focus have these same kinds of experiences.

Love is more than just romantic feelings between two people. It is our relationship to all of our experience and to the whole world. But many cultures, and many in our culture, regard the world as a place "out there," a dangerous or sinister place to be feared or exploited. We objectify the world rather than merge with it. If we learn to change the way we attend, our relationship with everything, including our planet, changes. We become part of the natural environment instead of apart from it, and develop a deeply rooted, heartfelt union with it. This is the all-encompassing, unconditional love described by Louisa in her letter at the beginning of the chapter. Can you imagine a world where we are all living in Open Focus, dissolving our pain, anxiety, restlessness, boredom, uncertainty, and ennui? Can you imagine freely giving and receiving love? Can you imagine also merging with the world instead of only objectifying it and feeling isolated and separate from it? Can you imagine sensing and experiencing the world as the wondrous place it can become and really is? These changes are very much within reach. It begins with the now-familiar question: How are you paying attention?

Exercise

Heart-Centered Open Focus

INTRODUCTION

THE HUMAN HEART is more than a mechanical pump that circulates blood throughout our body. With forty thousand neurons and an electrical field many times stronger than that produced by the brain, the heart can be said to have a powerful intelligence of its own. The heart's elaborate network of neurons and neurotransmitters enables it to act independently of the brain. Some researchers believe that the heart can learn, remember, and produce feelings on its own.[1] Emotional information sent from the heart to the brain has profound effects on higher brain functions, influencing our perceptions, thought processes, health, learning abilities, and especially our ability to feel compassion and empathy.

Anger, anxiety, and depression stress the heart and are significant factors for heart disease.[2] The notion of emotional pain leaving us with a "broken heart" seems to be true in a literal as well as metaphorical sense. Because of physiological connections between the brain and the heart, brain synchrony is as important to heart health as it is to brain health. The heart-centered Open-Focus exercise is reported to help the heart recover from stress. Individuals, couples, and groups can benefit from practicing this heart-centered Open-Focus exercise.

PREPARATION QUESTIONS

Can you imagine sitting gently upright and balancing yourself over your hips with your eyes closed?

Can you imagine that your imagination happens freely and effortlessly?

Can you imagine that distance and volume are experienced the same way as space: like the space between your fingers, like the space your fingers occupy?

Can you imagine centering your foreground attention upon feeling and especially upon the feeling of space while including other sense experiences and their space in the surround or background of your attention?

Can you imagine centering your attention upon the feeling of space surrounding and penetrating through available feeling sensations?

Can you imagine that initially you may only be able to narrow focus upon the feeling of one body space at a time as mentioned in this exercise?

Can you imagine that with continued practice your attention will broaden with each question, adding together your separate experiences of the individual body spaces into a feeling of one whole space?

Can you imagine what it would feel like if you were already feeling the presence of your whole body while feeling the space your body occupies and the space around and through your body?

GUIDING QUESTIONS

Can you imagine what it would feel like if you were already feeling the presence of your heart and the space it occupies and the space around and through your heart?

Can you imagine feeling the location of your heart within the space your body occupies?

Can you imagine what it would be like to feel the space between your heart and your breastbone?

Can you imagine feeling the space between your heart and your backbone?

Is it possible for you to imagine feeling the space between your heart and your throat and mouth?

Can you imagine feeling the distance between your heart and the space inside your stomach?

Can you imagine feeling the space between your heart and each of your ribs on both sides of your chest?

Is it possible for you to imagine what it would be like to feel the distance between your heart and the space inside your nose, your sinuses, your throat, your windpipe, and your lungs?

Can you imagine feeling the distance between your heart and the space inside your mouth, your throat, your stomach, and lower digestive system?

Can you imagine the space between your heart and your waist?

Can you imagine the space between your heart and the region between your navel and your backbone?

Can you imagine what it would be like to feel the space between your heart and the region occupied between your middle and lower spine?

Can you imagine the space between your heart and the region between your hips?

Is it possible for you to imagine the space between your heart and your buttocks, upper legs, knees, lower legs, ankles, feet, and toes?

Can you imagine the space between your heart and the region under your arms?

Can you imagine the space between your heart and your shoulders, upper arms, elbows, wrists, hands, and fingers?

Can you imagine what it would be like to experience the space flowing through your heart and the space flowing through the soles of your feet and the palms of your hands, all simultaneously?

Can you imagine what it would feel like to experience the space between your heart and your shoulder blades?

Can you imagine the space between your heart and your lips, tongue, teeth, gums, and the space inside your mouth and cheeks?

Can you imagine the space between your heart and the region between your cheeks?

Can you imagine the space between your heart and your jaw?

Can you imagine the distance between your heart and the space inside your ears, and the space between your ears?

Can you imagine the distance between your heart and the region of space inside and between your temples?

Can you imagine the distance between your heart and the region of space inside and between your eyes?

Can you imagine the space between your heart and your eyelids, eyebrows, and your forehead?

Can you imagine the space between your heart and the back of your head and the top of your head and the sides of your head?

Can you imagine the space between your heart and your whole head and face?

Can you imagine the space between your heart and the air touching your skin all over your body?

Can you imagine what it would be like to feel the sense of presence of your heart as a cloud of atoms floating in space, a space that extends in every direction and as far as you can imagine?

Is it possible for you to imagine what it would feel like to experience the space around your heart as continuous with the space through the cloud of atoms that is your heart?

Can you imagine the distance between the location of your feeling awareness itself and the location of your heart?

Can you imagine that the cloud of feeling awareness and the cloud of atoms that is your heart float toward each other and become one feeling experience, one combined cloud of awareness, space, and heart?

Is it possible for you also to imagine that any emotions or other body feelings that are currently present are also experienced as clouds of feeling floating in space?

Can you imagine now that these clouds of emotion and other feelings also combine with the clouds of your awareness and heart floating in space?

Is it possible for you now to imagine the space that flows through each of your other senses—visualizing, hearing, tasting, smelling, thinking, and a sense of time?

Can you imagine that these clouds of sensation also merge with the clouds of awareness, space, and heart?

Can you imagine opening your eyes and also including seeing in your heart-centered attention without interfering in any way with your broadened present attention?

Please now open your eyes. Can you imagine seeing through objects and space and bringing this visual experience into your heart-centered Open-Focus attention?

Can you imagine what it would be like for space to diffuse in every direction through your heart-centered multisensory attention?

Exercise

> Can you imagine engaging in daily activities while centered in your heart in Open Focus, paying attention to all objects and space that are available to you, effortlessly and simultaneously?
>
> Can you imagine practicing this exercise at least twice daily?

8

Peak Performance

Anything worth doing is
worth doing effortlessly.

— ANONYMOUS

THOMAS'S PASSION was playing trumpet. He played for Broadway plays and in dinner theaters; his real love, however, was jazz and blues, and he played in various bands around New York's lively club scene. But as he got older he noticed that performing made him more anxious. Every new gig meant a fresh audition; and sometimes, as he waited to stand up for a solo, the anxiety was almost overwhelming, which took a toll on the quality of his performance.

Thomas became a client and was diagnosed with performance anxiety and attention deficit disorder. Working with Open-Focus exercises both at home and in our office, he devised an exercise for himself: As he sat in front of the neurofeedback equipment, Thomas imagined he was in an audition or performance. "You're onstage now—go!" he told himself as the light and sound feedback were presented to him. Instead of concentrating more intently and trying harder, though,

Thomas learned from the feedback to relax his effort, open the scope of his attention, and merge with his anxiety and tension while he was performing.

He was surprised to find out just how uptight he was. As the light and sound feedback came on and he learned what it felt like to let go, his muscles relaxed, his anxiety diminished, and his music started to change. His self-consciousness disappeared, his playing was more spontaneous, and his jazz improvisations felt looser and more creative. He connected better with the drummer and bass player and, as he puts it, "I could be more in the moment, which is what good music is all about." But the training didn't just relax him; it also enhanced the sense of presence that a good performance requires. In addition, he was very surprised that a chronic rash on his hand, which often worsened when work was demanding, cleared up.

Few people would seem to be less in need of attention training than professional musicians, world-class athletes, and the like. "Seem" is the operative word here, for even someone who is at the top of their game can benefit—sometimes a great deal—from removing physical and emotional blockages through the appropriate use of flexible attention, which most often means shifting their attention when narrow focus is not required. Many high-functioning people have the idea that the harder they push, the better they will perform. But that is often not the case. Rather, everyone needs to know when to push hard and when not to, when to narrow focus and when to use diffuse or other styles of attention. Those who perform only in narrow focus are often "hyper-focused" and waste much energy fighting their own tense, overly excited physiology, which further increases muscle tension and raises heart and respiratory rates. These problems often worsen during competition, when focus narrows even further.

Narrow focus also engenders performance anxiety. When a baseball player suddenly can't throw to second base, a golfer can't putt without hitting the ball too hard, or a piano player can't relax enough to play a piece with feeling, it's in part because they are trying so hard—are so intent in their narrow focus—that they can't even consider diffusing and, as a result, seize up to some degree.

When the great cellist Pablo Casals was very old he could barely walk. Someone had to help him to his chair on the stage and prop the cello between his legs. But once he began to play, his true nature seemed to reappear as the bow flew across the strings with vigor and grace. How do you think he was able to overcome his physical limitations?

A woman I know who plays the piano had been struggling to play a Mozart sonata. She hadn't heard of Open Focus, and I suggested she listen to an exercise. "At first I couldn't stand the flute music that plays behind the exercise," she said. (I often play this flute music in the background when I introduce a person to Open Focus.) "Then I got into it and I found it very compelling. It felt like an extraordinarily deep meditation session." She went on:

> My body unwound itself. I had sat down on my piano bench, because it is good for maintaining a relaxed, correct posture. When I opened my eyes, at the close of the tape, I was looking at a Mozart sonata I'd been struggling with. I started playing, maintaining open focus as instructed, and I was amazed to find that passages that had intimidated me just flew effortlessly off my fingers.

The ability to flexibly attend, in fact, is one of the primary factors that make the difference between a good musician and a great musician—or athlete or student or corporate executive.

Attention and Synchrony Are How We Increase Flow

As they fixed arrows to bowstrings, a team of championship archers at Arizona State University had their EEG monitored. How, researchers wondered, do the brains of peak athletes function during performance? Dr. Dan Landers, a professor of physiology at ASU, found that when an archer is mentally preparing to shoot, the brain is chattering away at 13 to 20 hertz, high-frequency activity within the beta range. Then, just before the arrow is launched, alpha rhythms (8–12 hertz) wash over the left hemisphere of these top archers, calming the brain and body, quieting the mental chatter, and allowing full yet fluid dedication to and immersion in the task.[1] Research shows that the EEG pattern is the same for high-caliber rifle shooting, pistol shooting, karate, golf putting, and basketball free-throw shooting.[2]

The problem is that moving out of desynchronized beta into synchronized alpha is a subtle shift; without training in, and an experience of this activity, it's difficult for people to evoke them. A fish in water, it's been said, doesn't know it's in water. People often fail to recognize that they are carrying tension, perhaps because it increases gradually and persists for so long. I've had clients tell me they are deeply relaxed even when measurements of their physiology show them to be very tense.

A client named Mark had been meditating for years but felt he hadn't gotten much out of it. Monitoring with neuro-feedback equipment showed that he was very desynchronized and tense, and had trouble relaxing into alpha. I asked him to meditate using his mantra. Again, he produced much tension and high-frequency desynchronized beta and little alpha. He stopped meditating, and I asked him to let the light and sound feedback increase, signaling the presence of whole-brain synchronous alpha. As he gradually got more feedback, he discovered what alpha synchrony felt like and realized that he had been trying too hard. Then I asked him to meditate in such a way that the light and sound came on more often. Within minutes he felt as if his mantra was flowing effortlessly. After years of trying to meditate, he learned the meaning of effortlessness in a single neurofeedback session. His pallid face became ruddy and his demeanor brightened, both changes reflecting his newly achieved harmony.

Dr. Landers and his graduate students were able to teach a similar skill to the archery team. They divided the archers into two groups—some who got biofeedback training to learn to increase alpha and others who got non-alpha training—sham feedback training that does not produce alpha—as a control. "Those who got the alpha biofeedback showed significant improvement," Landers says. "Their shots moved from the outer edge of the nine ring to the inner. For archers that's a meaningful change." Those who received the non-alpha feedback did not improve.[3]

MUSCLE MEMORY

A major element of any performance, from singing to pole vaulting, is the baseline level of tension of the body's muscles. Muscles and muscle groups are almost never completely at rest. Some electrical firing of muscle cells is needed to maintain the structural alignment, posture, and balance of the body. Ideally, however, muscle tone is kept to a minimum so that when the body is called on for a task, the muscle system will be able to distribute the workload in a flexible and coordinated way. The ability to diffuse one's attention equally throughout the body is key.

Most of us, however, are unwittingly clunking around in a kind of body armor, our muscles habitually tensed because of chronic defensive reactions to emotional or physical trauma. Tense muscles force other muscles to compensate, which greatly hampers fluid performance. Unconsciously held muscle tension requires sympathetic autonomic activation, yielding anxiety, increased heart rate, and drained energy resources, leading to depression.

Open Focus works on a couple of levels for performers. Long-term attention training—lasting weeks or months—facilitates a deep release of chronic muscle tension, which improves coordination and stamina. This release is extraordinarily complete, much deeper than massage, stretching, or using heat. As training progresses, moving in and out of Open Focus becomes a familiar experience. Athletes can feel looser and less tense instantly by varying attention in the moment. Open Focus can be engaged while running, getting into starting blocks, waiting for a football to be snapped, stepping up to the free-throw line, drawing a bowstring, or sighting a target.

FROM GOLF TO KARATE TO FOOTBALL

Just as they grip the club with their hands, golfers grip the ball with their attention. Many subconsciously think gritting their teeth and bearing down will improve their game, but the opposite is true. Different styles of attention are needed for different parts of the game, and golfers can learn to move into the style of attention appropriate for a particular aspect of play. Fifteen or twenty minutes of Open-Focus exercises before a round loosens muscles. Placing the ball on the tee and getting ready to drive calls for the strategic mind of narrow focus; one must assess the lie of the holes, the direction and force of the wind, the wetness of the fairway and green, and the location of trees and traps, as well as other variables. A more diffuse and immersed focus helps integrate this information and loosen muscles for a few practice swings. Moving into Open Focus for the back swing immediately relaxes major muscle groups and facilitates a full and fluid downswing.

In narrow focus a golfer's attention is almost exclusively on the ball. By contrast, in Open Focus the center of attention of the player gently rests on the ball but at the same time admits a simultaneous and effortless awareness of things within peripheral attention—the sight of the grass, the trees, other features of the landscape, and the space in which sensations occur. There is an awareness of the scent of the grass, the sound of birds, and the feel of the club handle. During the swing the golfer's awareness diffuses and merges into an even fuller oneness with experience—all the while keeping attention centered on the ball—to the point that many report that their sense of self disappears.

Open-Focus training is not just about relaxation but also helps to optimize an athlete's physical resources, even for events that require a great deal of physical force. As a certified "speed-and-explosion" coach, I know that the ability to quickly accelerate from rest to top speed is essential to everything from football to basketball, racket sports, and track events. Most speed-training specialists use direct training strategies—pacing running players with a car moving just a little faster than their previous top speed or using electronic metronomes that click at a slightly faster beat than a player's usual footfall rate. But attention training, whether used by itself or in conjunction with other approaches, can also play a critical role in enhancing athletic performance.

I worked with Bob Ward, then the conditioning coach of the Dallas Cowboys. He traveled to Princeton for a few days of intensive training in Open Focus. Each morning Ward did his

119

usual stretches and calisthenics, taking up to two hours to loosen his muscles and ease his chronic lower-back and joint pain. After watching his exercises, I suggested doing some Open Focus in place of the usual conditioning routine. Within twenty minutes, I had guided Ward into Open Focus and through the dissolving-pain exercise, which quickly reduced his muscle tension and chronic pain. Ward was a convert and later asked me to introduce Open Focus to the Dallas Cowboys players and to a national conference of speed-and-explosion coaches.

RUNNING IN OPEN FOCUS

In preparation for the 1980 Olympics the U.S. Olympic Development Committee asked me to conduct performance enhancement sessions at the University of Illinois in Urbana-Champaign with twenty-two world-class runners who excelled at middle- and long-distance events. The runners spent three days training in Open Focus and using biofeedback instruments to measure muscle tension, sweat-gland activity, body-surface temperature, and brain-wave activity.

After being introduced to Open-Focus training, one runner at the session recounted how he had discovered an open style of attention on his own. One day he felt mildly ill at a track meet and didn't feel like running. But he entered the race anyway. After the starter's pistol sounded he dropped back in the pack to avoid the jostling, and ran last for a while. This was not, he thought, going to be his best run. Along with his ill feelings, however, he noticed he was starting to slip into what seemed like an altered state. He was simultaneously aware of the symptoms of his illness, the sound of his footfalls on the cinder track, the wind on his face, and other sensations he usually ignored. His effortful, goal-oriented focus fell away, and his internal monologue quieted. At the two-thirds point in the race he thought that if he was going to have a shot at winning the race he would have to "kick" into a sprint pretty soon. Then it happened, but without his having to exert extra effort. He was loose and suddenly found himself running so fast that he won the race in record time.

He had experienced a spontaneous Open-Focus attention shift. Subsequent attention training made the feeling much more familiar to him and easier to access.

Other Open-Focus trainees experience their sport in a more intuitive way, and physiological measurements reflect some of these changes. Dr. Lester Ingber, a physicist and a karate instructor with a fourth-degree black belt from the Japanese Karate Association, told me that by maintaining a "center of focus in his abdomen," just below his navel, he could rest within a diffuse, all-around readiness. Whenever an opponent made a move, Ingber felt his own broadened energy and awareness converge instantly on that center of focus like a broad beam of light focused through a lens. His focused, involuntary response emanated from this center. Then his centered attention spread out again.

In an experiment I conducted, Dr. Ingber was wired to EEG equipment. When he accessed his diffuse readiness the recordings showed low-frequency brain-wave synchrony, usually in the alpha range. The trigger to measure his reaction time was the sound of a loud click. Every time he heard the click, Ingber reacted by pressing a switch. He would generate alpha brain waves of 10 hertz while waiting for the click. When his reaction times were fastest, he would generate brain waves that were multiples of 10, so the response might be at 20, 30, and even 40 hertz or more. Then Ingber would return quickly to his poised and open attention. This is flexible attention.

121

By not narrow-objective focusing on any one stimulus, Ingber could open his awareness to the whole of his opponent's rhythm and react spontaneously in far less time than it would take for the execution of voluntary action. Ingber calls this "cutting his opponent's rhythm." It is as if he can slow the perceived motion of his opponent's actions and respond to them at a faster rate.

PERCEPTUAL CHANGES

In addition to improving endurance and reaction time and contributing to effortless performance, flexible attention also often impacts sensory experience. A New York jogger I worked with ran in Open-Focus attention. One day he emerged from Central Park to find his distance vision surprisingly sharpened and magnified. His adjustments to the path, the traffic, and other joggers had been quicker and more intuitive; these reactions had seemed to occur without thought or effort.

Some athletes say they have unusual perceptual experiences during performance. Baseball hitters I've trained say they can sometimes effortlessly see the path, position, and details of a pitched baseball, which appears to be coming toward them in slow motion. Or a soccer goalie sees the ball hang almost motionless on its trajectory toward him through the air. Some say they often perceive high-speed action in slow motion, and some see spontaneously shifting foreground and background.

These perceptions are functions of attention. Diffuse and immersed styles of attention are associated with phase-synchronous alpha states, in which people tend to perceive events as simultaneous, timeless, and all-inclusive. One psychiatrist who studied Open Focus had played college football and saw similarities between his experiences in Open Focus and his experiences of slowed time during episodes of peak performance on the football field. He had a "sixth sense" of where the ball and players had been, where they were in the present, and where they were going to be in the future.

"Keep your eye on the ball." Generations of tennis instructors have used this adage, and their students have paid the price. As with any object of attention, narrow focus on the ball in tennis produces tension. By contrast, Open-Focus training encourages players to center on the ball while being simultaneously and effortlessly aware of everything on the court. Players find that their perception and creativity are unlocked, along with a feeling of effortless play, when they include an awareness of peripheral, or background, details. This also enhances three-dimensional experience; as the tennis ball hurtles in your direction, it's more visually prominent and seems to materialize out of its three-dimensional surroundings.

An example of how narrow focus limits our perception, and how attentional flexibility can unlock it, is seen in the story of an avid sport climber named Jerry. Under a jutting overhang on a craggy peak in Colorado, his climb suddenly grew difficult. Isolated from his companion on a rock cliff far above the ground, Jerry was overcome by panic and in this agitated state couldn't find handholds or footholds. He tried to tamp down the rising anxiety by focusing more intently on his climbing, but he remained immobilized.

Seeing him in trouble, Jerry's companion shouted to him, "Remember Open Focus!" Hands trembling, Jerry started opening his awareness, taking in his peripheral attention. After a few minutes his mind started to clear, his body relaxed, his hands stopped shaking, and he became flexible again. His panic subsided, his grip seemed sure, and he felt connected with the mountain. Everywhere he looked, it seemed, there were notches for handholds and footholds. After a few minutes in Open Focus, with his outlook greatly improved, he easily climbed on and finished his ascent.

OPEN FOCUS TAKES THE STAGE

Performance coach Rae Tattenbaum coaches young singers at the highly regarded Hartt School of Music in West Hartford, Connecticut, where she is on the faculty of the Department of Voice and Theater. Tattenbaum benefited from Open Focus herself and began using it to train performers. Her young singers are classically trained and will someday audition for entrance into college music departments. They've received excellent technical training and know how to hit a note by supporting the tone with the diaphragm; however, they're often anxious and therefore not fully present—physically or emotionally—when they perform. Tattenbaum's goal is to enable the singers to become completely absorbed in a free and spontaneous performance.

Peak performers in any field are often people who are genetically blessed with the ability to move in and out of synchrony. I have observed that good actors, for example, move into synchrony when they are acting, allowing the role they are playing to subsume their own identity. Otherwise it seems as if they are faking it.

An actor once called me and asked if I could train him to stay immersed in his role. He had no problem getting into his roles, but staying in them was more difficult. I suggested that instead of trying to stay in a role, he should learn to quickly reenter it, which is a function of flexible attention.

Tattenbaum uses a number of approaches in her work, including several weeks of special Open-Focus exercises she devised to release the face and throat muscles as well as the groin and diaphragm. "All of my singers have this gripping in

124

their facial mask, and they have to let it go," she says. "Once they use attention training to release face muscles, and open their focus, their whole physiology responds and releases. They can better employ the diaphragm. They feel like they own their space on stage, and they can use their performance muscles the way they were meant to be used."

Tattenbaum created her own Open-Focus exercises to help the singers let go of everything from past trauma to audition jitters, allowing them to truly and deeply release. They are trained to expand their awareness during performance, to include the other singers and musicians, the members of the audience, all of the motion and other sensory elements in the theater, and the space and silence in which they occur.

At their most open and uninhibited, Tattenbaum says, performers intuitively shift their physical energies and take their voices to new levels. "Open Focus allows people to harness power to perform that I have not seen before," she says. "Once you have begun the 'seeding' process, that is, once you've taught them Open Focus and they get it and it becomes second nature, they own their power. You have given them quite a gift."

Singers who train with Open-Focus exercises, she says, have better range, the colors in their voices are richer, and they are better able to get in touch with the emotion of the piece they are performing. Robin, a singer and teacher at Hartt, says: "I noticed I couldn't be present as a performer. I used to feel like I was outside myself, watching and judging. The training gave me an overall sense of well-being that I didn't have before. I can step back, take a breath, and focus on and merge with my performance much better."

The best studies on brain-wave training and the performance of musicians have been done by Dr. Jonathan Gruzelier, at the Imperial College London, with musicians from the Royal College of Music in London.

Nearly a hundred students were given different types of neurofeedback training. Those who received an alpha/theta protocol improved their performance the most. The alpha/theta group improved their performance between 13.5 and 17 percent. Dr. Gruzelier said, "These results show that neurofeedback can have a marked effect on musical performance. While it has a role in stress reduction by reducing the level of stage fright, the magnitude and range of beneficial effects on artistic aspects of performance have wider implications than alleviating stress."[4]

9

Living in Open Focus

To infinity and beyond!

— Buzz Lightyear
in *Toy Story*

S EVERAL YEARS ago I went to a local amusement park in hopes of conquering a lifelong fear of heights. On a ride called Free Fall I sat in a small cage and was slowly hoisted up twenty stories. As I looked out at 360 degrees of New Jersey farmland I desperately wanted to be somewhere else. My palms grew sweaty, my hands gripped a bar in front of me, my legs quivered, and a painful anxious feeling welled up in the pit of my stomach and chest as I got farther above the ground. The cage dangled for a few seconds that seemed to last an eternity; then a loud buzzer sounded and the cage suddenly plummeted fifteen stories before slowing to a stop at the bottom. I was absolutely terrified, my hands shook, and after the ride every muscle in my body seemed to remain tense.

My second ride took place in Open Focus. As I waited in line and as the cage was hoisted, I searched out the physical location of my fear and found it in my stomach and chest. Instead of bracing against these feelings, I put myself fully in touch with them. I broadened my awareness, becoming aware of background as well as foreground. I accessed all of my senses simultaneously—seeing, hearing, feeling, smelling, and tasting sense objects near and far, as well as the space that permeated and surrounded them.

I experienced the space around and inside of me and imagined myself as a cloud of particles floating in and permeated by a vast space. I moved toward and relaxed into the fear-driven pain in my stomach and chest. Almost immediately my muscles relaxed and the knot of fear started to subside. By the time the cage reached its peak, the fear and tension were gone.

The cage dropped. But this time I remained surprisingly calm. I soon recognized the reason for the change. In my first attempt, I had braced myself against the trembling and other manifestations of fear. But this very act of trying to ward off my feelings had amplified a set of simple physical sensations into an experience of terror. However, when I opened myself to the actual sensory experiences at hand and to an awareness of the space surrounding and suffusing them, the situation no longer felt like an emergency.

It is in this paradoxical way that narrow focus can bring about precisely the experiences we seek to avoid and Open Focus can free us from them. In narrow focus, we resist our experience but stay riveted to an exaggerated version of it. In Open Focus, by contrast, we allow our experience while inviting our underused senses, including that of space, to surround and diffuse it. A life lived in flexible attention changes everything. Daily life is more effortless, from waking up and getting dressed to eating, driving, working, studying, enjoying our family relationships, undertaking creative endeavors, and competing in sports. It changes the way we anticipate the future and remember the past. We become more relaxed and less anxious; we sleep better and are more loving. We allow emotions to be experienced and diffused effortlessly, instead of letting our emotions generate resistance and overreaction. Internal negative criticism gives way to a light, clear mind, an inner calm. Problems seem to present their own solutions, relationships of all kinds become more engaging, and the world becomes a friendlier place.

LEARNING IN OPEN FOCUS

Open Focus has obvious implications for learning. Without anxiety we can pay attention longer and with less effort and distraction. Distinction between styles of attention, fluid and relevant figure-ground processing, and timing of style application are critical factors for all learning.

The human brain is divided into right and left hemispheres. While older studies showed a distinct difference between the right and left brain, more recent studies show things are more complex. But it's still clear that each half has responsibility for different functions. The right brain expresses emotions and perceives facial signals, coordinates singing, comprehends music, reads body language and body awareness, and carries out visual-spatial tasks needed to throw and catch a ball or ride a bike. It facilitates insight and intuitive reasoning and immersion, for example, in the experience of three-dimensional space and three-dimensional spatial relationships. The right brain takes in the big picture and context, in both a literal and a metaphorical sense, seeing many things simultaneously rather than in sequence. This is called parallel processing. It perceives a whole face at once, for example, rather than individual

129

features one at a time. Familiarity and recognition are right-brain functions.

The left brain, on the other hand, is the dominant hemisphere in our culture, generally more objective, separate, and rational than emotional, with a strong positive sense of self.[1] It governs language, speech, reading, writing, and sequential, or serial, information processing, which includes such tasks as understanding grammar, doing arithmetic, typing, and keeping score, all of which are made possible through the use of narrow-objective attention.

The differences between the left and right hemispheres of the brain were first systematically studied in people who had had them separated surgically as a last resort to eliminate seizures. In these subjects it was found that an object seen only by the left eye and conveyed only to the right brain can be recognized but not named because the left brain, concerned with naming, is out of the loop. When seen only by the right eye and conveyed only to the left brain, the same object can be named but not recognized, because the right brain is missing from the mix. Similarly, the right hemisphere, which is responsible for music, can recognize the melody of a song but not its lyrics, while the left hemisphere, with its emphasis on language, can recall a song's words but has no memory of its melody. Although people who have not undergone this surgery do not exhibit such overt split-brain phenomena, we all have a dominant hemisphere, much as we are either right-handed or left-handed. Right-brained individuals tend to be creative, with a broader, "big-picture," diffuse-immersed type of attention; they are less concerned about details such as time and deadlines and balancing their checkbook. Artists, performers, and those dealing with imagination and invention are more inclined to be right brained. Left brainers are usually more narrowly and objectively focused, with rigid, goal-oriented attitudes.

We live in a society born of the left hemisphere—two-thirds of the population are left-brain dominant. Many occupations and most males favor left-brain function. Our culture—as embodied in our schools, workplaces, government, and military—is left-brain biased. These institutions are concerned with written language, time, deadlines, serial processing, objects, and an outward, objective focus. They reward left-hemisphere dominant people and marginalize those with right-hemisphere dominance. The result is a society that is materially rich but impoverished in many important ways.

To function at its best, human consciousness must blend the attention functions of the right and left hemispheres. Narrow-objective focus is the province of the left brain, while diffuse-immersed is the province of the right. We call the optimal blend Open Focus, an unbiased state in which all types of attention are present more or less equally. As I've mentioned, our society's balance of attention styles is generally tipped in favor of left-hemisphere processing. One way we can correct this imbalance is to practice attention exercises—such as those included in this book—involving space, volume, and other stimuli that activate the right hemisphere.

One of the big questions in the study of the brain is the binding question: How does the brain bring its disparate regions together to create a consciousness that contains many perceptions simultaneously? Synchrony is key, which is mediated by attention. Learning an open style of attention generates synchronous alpha in the major lobes of the brain; this reduces stress and allows fluid communication among different regions of the brain, improving mental function effortlessly and naturally. The complex, carefully timed nature of brain function has been compared to a symphony orchestra. But a brain that works only in narrow-objective focus is like an orchestra trying to play from the lyrics and an absent or incomplete score; the music doesn't sound as it should. Fully flexible attention brings all lobes of the brain fully online and restores them to a harmonious relationship, creating a symphony of conscious experience. This has implications for everything we do, especially learning.

There are some disorders that research shows are, at least in part, a malfunction of the brain's timing mechanisms, including Down syndrome, mental retardation, and even autism. These problems can potentially respond well to neurofeedback. In an unpublished pilot study one of my colleagues, Dr. Geri Fee, academically trained six children with Down syndrome when brain synchrony feedback was presented and not otherwise. Dr. Fee performed the training and school psychologists performed pre- and post-IQ testing. Before the study the children's IQs ranged from 40 to 47. After several months of academic and alpha synchrony training, the children made impressive gains, raising their IQ to between 81 and 87, which is considered "slow normal."

A number of researchers believe that autism is a problem of how the brain binds together different sites to coordinate consciousness, thus suggesting a functional rather than a structural problem. In one study at the University of Washington, researchers studied alpha waves, simply asking people to close their eyes and then measuring the EEG. They found that in the group of people with autism, the communication between different regions of the brain was diminished, particularly in the frontal lobes, which are responsible for socialization, one of the key aspects of autism. The answer, according to Dr. Marcel Just, a researcher at Carnegie Mellon University, is in changing the timing. "One can imagine also training or therapies that are designed to teach the various parts of the brain to work together in a more coordinated way, to make them function as a team instead of individual players," Just told National Public Radio.*

In one study that's what we did. Two colleagues and I trained an eight-year-old boy with autism. After thirty-one sessions of training, the boy showed positive changes in all diagnostic categories that define autism. He warmed up emotionally and "for the first time in his life he played with his sister, and even kissed her, and put his arm around his older brother."† This has profound implications for a disorder with few therapeutic options. That is, if controlled experiments confirm these findings.

However, in our culture most initial learning depends on paying attention exclusively in a serial way—that is, in narrow-objective focus—moving from point to point, movement to movement, or process to process. Checking off items one by one on a to-do list is a typical example of serial processing. In this goal-oriented process, attention narrows so as to tightly grasp its object and to prevent anything else from causing distraction.

Most public education in our culture also stops with serial processing. Although this style of learning is valuable, different kinds of learning require different attention styles. For example, the diffuse-immersed style of attention is more appropriate for music, art, acting, and other skills that depend on parallel processing. However, even left-brain tasks profit from being done with a more open style of attention. Subtle patterns become perceptible, seeming to jump out from the

* *All Things Considered,* October 17, 2006.
† "Positive Outcome with Neurofeedback Treatment in Case of Mild Autism," Arthur G. Sichel, Lester G. Fehmi, and David M. Goldstein, *Journal of Neurotherapy,* Summer 1995.

background. When one has greater scope and immersion of attention, creative problem solving in every context—social, academic, professional, and athletic—is facilitated.

A FLEXIBLE-ATTENTION LIFESTYLE

The multidimensional awareness that Open Focus brings can be used for almost anything, whether something we have done before or something new we are learning. Take the components of tennis—timing the swing with the oncoming ball, serving the ball, getting the right racket alignment, using the right amount of force; all of these benefit from narrow-objective focus. But the game also requires parallel processing, the coordinated use of the whole body, as well—planting the feet and bringing the racket back at the same time, for example. Optimal play seldom occurs when we try to narrow focus on one task and then another. But when we incorporate multiple styles of attention to process the various tasks in parallel—for example, simultaneously staying aware of three-dimensional space and background, the location of our opponent, and running for the ball—there's an effortless integration, a smooth execution that allows us to get out of our own way.

Playing music in a band works the same way. A musician has to hear all of the sounds of other instruments and blend his own sound in. That means serially processing his own playing and simultaneously listening to the music of others in diffuse attention. If he is very good, he can engage the witnessing process, which hovers above all the individual performances and perceives them as an integrated whole.

During sex there is a time when narrow focus on sensual stimuli is appropriate—it fans desire. If you stay narrowly focused on one aspect—the other person as a sexual object, for instance—it may be pleasant, but it limits the richness of the encounter and blocks a fuller and richer experience, one that extends beyond the sexual organs and even the body itself. For this, Open-Focus attention is needed. Open Focus makes it possible to merge fully with the other person and to witness and enter the whole experience at once. This takes sex out of the realm of the merely sensual and makes it also transcendent and sacred.

When we approach our jobs with the right balance of attention styles, our work improves and becomes more effortless. One day as I walked down a street in Little Tokyo in Los Angeles, I watched a man repeatedly pour batter for thirty pancakes on a grill in the front window of a bean-cake factory. He worked quickly but not hurriedly, maintaining a steady rhythm that made pouring batter and cooking pancakes seem effortless. In every occupation there are people who have found their own way—consciously or unconsciously—to a combination of attention styles that makes their work easier and less stressful. But in a society so dominated by narrow-objective focus, this is not something that comes naturally to most of us. With Open-Focus training, the process of finding the right balance of attention styles is no longer left to chance but is engaged intentionally.

DAILY LIFE IN OPEN FOCUS

Narrow-focus habits are so entrenched in most of us that we may easily forget to use Open Focus during the day. Even if you practice the exercises included in this book daily, with the goal of transferring the skills to the rest of your life activities, you may find yourself forgetting to do so. Even a few moments after completing a practice session, you may find yourself back in narrow-objective attention. Open Focus, while easy to do, can be hard to remember. After all, our practiced bias of narrow focus has taken many years, and each day it is reinforced. We need to remind ourselves to open our focus. But how can we do this?[2]

When uncomfortable emotions and physical sensations arise in daily life, we can take them as a reminder to open our awareness. Negative feelings are messages and should not be avoided or pushed away. Attempting to do so usually makes us more tense and in the long run just makes the feelings more intense. Somewhat ironically, the first step toward dissolving unpleasant experiences is to be with them and accept them into a simultaneous awareness of peripheral sensations and of space. The painful feelings will lessen and can often dissolve altogether.

Anything can be used as a cue to practice Open Focus. Some people find it helpful to place stickers or Post-It notes around their home or workplace as reminders. Whether you're waiting for the person you're calling to answer the phone, exercising, standing in line, sitting at a red light, cleaning, walking, or bathing, you can take advantage of the opportunity to broaden your attention.

There are daily, on-the-spot exercises that can help us to cultivate and maintain Open Focus. One of the habitual narrow-focus things we do, for example, is to identify a single object as the figure and relegate everything else around it to the background. We focus on a vase in a room, for example, but ignore the walls and furniture and carpet, which make up the background. The act of selecting and concentrating on one object out of a field of objects requires a lot of energy. Simply learning to shift what we consider figure and what ground, and being able to view them with equal interest, dramatically reduces effort and shifts the brain waves we produce and the way we think and feel.

Using the following technique daily, we can learn to maintain Open Focus anywhere—whether riding on the subway or sitting at the computer—simply by admitting into consciousness the space, silence, and timelessness that pervades our experience.

Whenever you think of it, carry out your everyday tasks while at the same time being aware of infinite space, silence, and timelessness. Be aware of the three-dimensional space between, around, and through objects. Attend to all your senses: seeing, hearing, feeling, taste, smell, mental activity, and time. Include both objects and space. Imagine an awareness of space that permeates everything. Imagine feeling the background space against which everything is highlighted.

When done in the midst of our everyday activities, this exercise quickly wakes up the right brain, opens our attention, and loosens the grip of the left brain on our experience of the world. With the activation of the right brain, the processes of perception, sensation, and imagination become more poignant and we find ourselves able to be more at ease, loving, and open. This engagement of the whole brain happens most readily when the four kinds of attention (narrow, diffuse, immersed, and objective) are used in a flexible and balanced way.

Positive and permanent change comes through practice. And just as we eventually learned to walk, ride a bike, throw a ball, or play piano without thinking about it, Open-Focus skills too can become automatic in our lives. Open-Focus training introduces people to their native, unself-conscious processes of attention, which may in fact have frequently been used before. But once awakened, these ways of being allow us to recognize the world, to feel at home in the world, and they are utterly natural.

137

APPLYING OPEN FOCUS

Professionals, coaches, and caregivers who have learned Open Focus often find ways to apply the technique in their own work. Antoinette, a massage therapist, uses objectless imagery for a few minutes to help herself relax before beginning a massage and to help her clients relax as well. When she finds a spasm or knot in the muscles, she presses in with her thumb and hand while having the client notice and pay attention to the quality and intensity of the pain. She asks the client a series of questions designed to help dissolve pain: "Can you feel the space around the pain? The space it occupies? Can you imagine allowing the space to permeate the pain as you accept and embrace the pain?" Massage, she says, is much more effective with guided Open-Focus questions.

An acupuncturist client of mine said he had trouble getting his patients to feel the *chi*, or subtle energy, moving through their bodies. After nine months of twice-daily Open-Focus practice, he wrote me in an e-mail: "I suddenly began to insert the needle differently and patients began to feel the chi moving through their body. I wanted to let you know that Open Focus has impacted not only my life but those of countless patients."

Teachers, physicians, psychotherapists, attorneys, mothers, fathers—anyone—can learn to be flexible in the way they pay attention. Applying Open Focus in daily life makes activities at home and work more fluid and effortless, and it models flexible attention to our families and colleagues.

Exercise

How Am I Now Paying Attention?

INTRODUCTION

THE KEY to learning to transfer Open-Focus awareness to everyday life is to stop and ask yourself "How am I now paying attention?" until that question grows to be second nature. The following questions are an inventory of the kinds of attention we need to learn to be aware of as we move into an Open Focus.

GUIDING QUESTIONS

How am I now paying attention?

Am I narrowly attending to visual objects and space?

Am I narrowly attending to hearing sounds and silence?

Am I narrowly attending to physical and emotional feelings and to feeling space?

Am I narrowly attending to smelling? And to tasting? And to the space in which they exist?

Am I narrowly attending to the internal silence in which internal dialogue occurs?

Am I narrowly attending to the space in which internal images occur?

Am I narrowly paying attention to my sense of nowness and timelessness, to my experience of this moment?

Which of these senses are present in my narrow and immersed awareness?

Can I imagine narrowly objectifying and at the same time diffusely merging with the space in which my sensations occur?

Can I melt into and merge with the mind space and mind silence in which internal dialogue occurs?

Can I become timelessness?

Can I pay attention to how I am paying attention at this moment?

How many senses are simultaneously available to me? And in how many senses is space available to me?

In which sensory modalities am I able to objectify and merge with the objects of sensation and the space within which they occur simultaneously?

In which sensory modalities am I able to narrow and diffusely attend to the objects of sensation and the space in which they occur simultaneously?

Can I imagine identifying the attention style within which I am resting, that is, while I am attending to how I am attending?

Can I imagine letting foreground and background freely interchange my attention of interest in each sense modality?

Can I imagine what it would be like if I were already in the habit of paying attention to how I pay attention?

Can I imagine what it would be like if I were already resting in the process of attending to how I am attending, more or less continuously?

10

Attention and Psychotherapy

The past is never dead.
It's not even past.

— WILLIAM FAULKNER,
Requiem for a Nun

I GENERALLY don't use talk therapy or deal with clients based on the content of their problems, but for some patients and some problems psychotherapy must be part of the treatment picture. My wife and longtime professional partner, Susan Shor Fehmi, MSW, has made an important original contribution in pioneering the integration of psychodynamic talk therapy with Open-Focus training. The material that follows is drawn from her experience and her views about how to blend the two approaches.

A client of hers named Gloria had progressed well in psychotherapy, having come to understand how her early feelings of helplessness in relation to her father still continued to affect her relationships with men, especially authority figures. She

knew intellectually that feeling helpless around men in authority was an echo of her past, and that knowledge helped her distance herself from the feelings. Yet she still experienced waves
of anxiety when the feelings of helplessness were stirred.

During one therapy session Gloria described an incident
with her boss. As she spoke to him, these feelings of helplessness started to rise in her, and she recognized in the moment
that these were really old childhood feelings. This helped her
to separate the past feelings from the present situation and kept
her from acting out with her employer in a neurotic way. As
she described to Susan the anxiety she felt during the incident,
however, the feelings of helplessness again reemerged. Susan
led her through an Open-Focus exercise that allowed her to
dissolve the feelings of helplessness and anxiety. Susan then
described to her how she might dissolve these feelings in the
"heat of battle."

Over time, Gloria became adept at dissolving these feelings
as they arose. Three months later, Gloria said the feelings of
helplessness rarely came up at work any more. When they did,
she could recognize that her attention had become overly narrow and objective. When she noticed narrow focus arising, she
diffused her attention, which in turn made it easy to immerse
herself in the feelings of helplessness until they dissolved.
Before long, Gloria could do this with all of her noxious feelings. Without Open Focus, psychotherapy would still have
helped Gloria to have a better life, but she would have been left
with painful feelings. In Susan's estimation, she became free of
chronic emotional pain faster using Open Focus than she
would have using talk therapy alone.

Attention plays a central but largely unacknowledged role
in talk therapy. Narrow-objective attention is the strategy we
use to repress unpleasant feelings and troublesome thoughts.
While alpha refers to a relaxed brain-wave activity, it also

corresponds to the type of attention in which we begin to open the door to repressed contents of the mind and to traumatic, emotionally charged memories of the past. Our typical reduction of alpha production, in other words, is a mechanism of repression. We reflexively produce more beta and less alpha in order to defend against noxious mental content becoming conscious. In her book *The High-Performance Mind*, Anna Wise, a veteran biofeedback therapist, calls alpha "the bridge to the unconscious."

THE ROLE OF ATTENTION IN EMOTIONAL HEALING AND GROWTH

Attention is central to the act of repression. The mind banishes unwanted emotional material by attending away from it in the same way that the mind can ignore a distracting noise by focusing away from it and turning its attention to something else. We use attention skills all the time to execute decisions about what to include and what to exclude from awareness.

We are so good at narrowly focusing our attention away from thoughts, feelings, and memories that we wish to avoid that we can often successfully keep them out of awareness for years and even permanently. This is successful repression, which is not all bad and can help us survive difficult emotional times. When repression is imperfect, however, and the repressed memories or feelings reemerge in our consciousness, we make the mistake of narrowly focusing away from them, trying to repress them again. It rarely works as well a second time, and the point at which repression stops holding back painful material is when people usually seek out psychotherapy.

Traditional psychotherapy attempts to allow the feelings and impressions emerging from the unconscious to find a home in our conscious mind through reliving painful situations, understanding, and insight. Analysis of dreams, slips of the tongue, humor, and free association are all psychodynamic tools that provide clues to the roots of noxious experiences such as anxiety. Once the sources are identified, understanding the painful experience and integrating it into conscious awareness often help the anxiety fade.

This therapeutic process, however, is also a form of attention training, for what is really happening in talk therapy is the gradual opening of attention and a melting into highly charged painful material that had been previously stored only in narrow-objective focus, keeping it at arm's length. But once admitted into consciousness, the heretofore repressed memories or emotions are integrated into here-and-now experience.

As a matter of fact, the processes of attention are at the center of psychotherapy, though it's seldom thought of that way. For instance, good psychotherapists intuitively understand the importance of moving clients into a more open, diffuse, and immersed style of attention, a shift that also has neurological effects, including the production of slower brain frequencies. Diffuse-immersed attention allows highly charged memories, which were stored during emergency events that elicited high-frequency brain activity, to surface in a state of lower arousal and be worked through.

Freud seems to have understood at some level the role attention plays in forming and releasing repressed thoughts and feelings. His patients would lie on a couch in a quiet, softly lit room, facing away from the therapist. They were encouraged to free-associate without self-editing and with very little input from him. They were asked to make no effort to concentrate attention in any way or toward anything in particular. Without distraction, patients could allow their thoughts and feelings to emerge and were encouraged to talk about them in

145

an uncensored and uninterrupted stream of consciousness. Perhaps Freud was helping his patients to develop a diffuse-immersed form of attention, one that allows emotional pain to become a smaller part of one's total awareness. When emotional pain is experienced within diffuse attention, it becomes easier to experience and makes us more willing to allow deeper, unexplored material to emerge.

All modern talk therapies use some form of this technique, which facilitates the gradual opening of a person's awareness, allows for the free emergence of feelings, and then provides methods of integrating those feelings. Psychotherapy, when it works long-term, changes the way we attend to our memories and feelings. We slowly open ourselves to them and come to terms with their powerful emotional charge. Moreover, a good therapist supports a de facto Open-Focus state in clients by modeling his attention process. Freud said he listened to his patients "with an evenly hovering attention."

In all forms of psychotherapy, attention plays an essential role in allowing material to come up and be integrated into conscious awareness. Open Focus training gives us a powerful tool we can use to merge with and dissolve those feelings, which reside not only in our memory but in our body as well.

For many of us, there's a habit of looking at content and ignoring process. We focus on the specific content of our emotional pain rather than looking at our attentional relationship to the pain itself—the way we tend to pull away and try to avoid it. A change in the way we attend to our pain is ultimately what helps us to live more contented and satisfying lives. When you start to look at process and content rather than just content alone, there's a paradigm shift and new attentional tools emerge.[1]

Put simply, excessive fixation, rigidity, obsession, repression, depression, resistance, detachment, loneliness, addiction, inhibition, neurosis, anxiety, and other reactions to the contents of attention are undermined with the development of flexible attention.

THE MARRIAGE OF OPEN FOCUS AND TALK THERAPY

At first Susan wasn't sure how to integrate Open Focus and psychotherapy—and neither was I. She felt obligated to provide psychotherapy clients with the kind of treatment they expected, and some clients have a real need to talk about the things they have done, felt, thought, and experienced in order to develop acceptance of painful material. At first we had a dual practice, using traditional talk therapy with some and Open-Focus training and neurofeedback with others.

After a while, Susan noticed that many Open-Focus clients began to spontaneously work through many of the same issues addressed in traditional psychotherapy. To her astonishment, they worked through them with greater ease and to a more complete resolution. Together we tentatively came up with a way of combining the two approaches. Susan discovered that using Open Focus with psychodynamic psychotherapy is a marriage made in heaven.

When a client's "big issues" have been successfully dealt with in talk therapy but some anxiety and other symptoms persist, switching to Open-Focus training (especially the dissolving-pain exercise) is very useful in quickly "cleaning up" what remains—for example, habitual gripping of the physical and emotional pain. This change of method has proven itself more efficient than talk therapy. Open Focus helps normalize physiology and accelerates the therapeutic process by making it easier for clients to accept the painful emotions stirred up in thoughts and memories. They find it easier to diffuse their attention and immerse themselves into painful feelings until they are dissolved. Furthermore, the whole process produces less anxiety because clients can now access a larger, more inclusive field of attention by merging with objects and with space, with no one thing occupying the whole of their attention. The anxiety becomes small stuff in a large field of awareness.

Open Focus takes a different view of emotional feelings in the body from that of the traditional psychotherapeutic approach, which sees them as "somatic displacement," a defense deployed to aid in the repression of the client's real emotions. Open Focus, on the other hand, regards the feelings as an integral part of the problem, searches them out in the body, and seeks to dissolve them.

The ability to immerse ourselves in pain while maintaining a diffuse attention is something we all need to learn to do in the heat of life's daily battles, but it is particularly useful in psychotherapy, where life's most difficult experiences are laid bare. Whether these are panic attacks, phobias, dysfunctional interpersonal patterns, or repressed thoughts, memories, and feelings, Open-Focus skills are a powerful way to reduce or eliminate them. Our personal and interpersonal lives can fundamentally change when we welcome these feelings and patterns into our awareness, knowing that we have a tool with which to dissolve them. Open Focus is the perfect place to start with any client. And in many cases, it is all that is necessary to bring about general well-being.

Exercise

Thinking in Open Focus

INTRODUCTION

NOWHERE IS the tenacious grip of narrow-objective focus more evident than in our relationship to thinking. We identify ourselves with the content of our thoughts, failing to realize that we are in fact something much greater: We are also the context in which thoughts arise. But in order to experience ourselves as such, we must first learn to be flexible in how we attend to thoughts. This exercise allows you to try out different ways of attending to thinking and its relationship with the other components of awareness—sensory perceptions, space, and time.

The process of thinking, which I consider a distinct sense, like seeing, hearing, or feeling, encompasses different types of mental contents. There is self-talk, or internal dialogue, which is what most people associate with the word "thinking." Additionally, we can mentally experience visual imagery that is current or remembered, created purely by imagination, or a combination of both. Feelings can drive or be present with the various forms of thinking. This is by no means an exhaustive list, but it's important to realize that the words "thinking" and "thoughts" in this exercise refer to turning one's attention to mental content. Also, when you are asked to identify the physical location from which thoughts seem to originate, please remember that such questions are designed to help you discover how you can release your experience of thinking at the body level, not to suggest that sophisticated information processing actually takes place at those particular sites.

Remember to allow fifteen seconds between questions.

PREPARATION
GUIDING QUESTIONS

Can you imagine centering your attention on your thoughts, whatever your thoughts are? Your thoughts might include visual images, feelings, self talk, or other types of perception.

Can you imagine that while you're centering your attention on thinking, you can remain aware of the space in which your thoughts occur? Your thoughts may be occurring in a visual space, or in a feeling space, or in silence. Your thoughts might be perceived as an internal voice— or a dialogue between internal voices—within silence.

Can you imagine centering your attention on thinking while simultaneously experiencing the space or silence in which thinking occurs?

At the same time that you're experiencing your thoughts, and centering your attention on the current location of your thoughts, and experiencing that mental space or silence in which your thoughts are occurring, can you imagine feeling the sense of presence of your whole body?

At the same time that you're centering your awareness on your thoughts and the space in which they occur, can you imagine feeling the sense of presence of your whole body, and, equally and simultaneously, the space around your body?

Can you imagine the free flow of thought in the space in which it occurs, while feeling body presence and emotions and the space in which they occur as background for thinking?

Can you imagine centering your attention on thinking, on the free flow of thought and the space in which thought occurs, and at the same time experiencing sounds, and the silence in which sounds occur, as a background for thought?

Can you imagine centering your attention on thinking and the mind-space in which thinking occurs and at the same time experiencing feeling and hearing and the space and silence in which they occur, as a background for thinking?

Can you imagine centering your awareness on the free flow of your thoughts in the space in which they occur and sensing taste and the space in which tastes occur as a background for thinking?

Can you imagine maintaining the center of your awareness on thoughts, on the free flow of thinking, while allowing taste and hearing and feeling to serve as a background for your thoughts?

Can you imagine centering your attention on thinking, on the space in which your thoughts arise, exist for a time, and diffuse, and allowing the sensation of smell, of whatever fragrances and odors are present, and its space, to serve as a background for thinking? Thoughts are figure; sensations of smell and the space in which they occur are background.

Can you imagine now including in the background also taste, sound, and feeling, and the background space in which these four sensations occur, while centering your attention on thinking as figure?

Can you imagine centering your attention on your thoughts and the space in which they occur and letting visual experience of space and objects serve as background to thinking?

Can you imagine now including also in the background smelling, tasting, hearing, and feeling, and the common space, silence, in which they occur, as you continue to center your attention on thinking and the flow of thought?

Can you imagine continuing to center your attention on thinking and the mind-space and mind-silence in which your thoughts occur, and now accepting a sense of time, a sense of nowness, a sense of present moment, and the timelessness in which this sense of time occurs, as background for thinking?

Can you imagine now including as part of the background for thinking also seeing, feeling, tasting, smelling, and hearing and the common background, silence, space, timelessness?

Can you imagine centering your attention on the location of your thoughts or thinking process in your body? Can you imagine feeling where in your body thinking occurs?

Can you imagine feeling where is the source of your thought? In your feet? In your legs? In your hands or arms? Do thoughts arise from a location in your lower trunk? Mid-trunk? Upper body? Neck? Face? Head? Where is the center of this thinking process located in your body?

Can you imagine continuing to center your awareness on your thoughts as you experience all your other sensations simultaneously, including the sense of presence of your whole body, and simply noticing where in your body space thoughts arise and exist for a time before they decay to make room for other thoughts?

Can you imagine centering your awareness on the flow of thought and simultaneously on the background sensations and space in which these thoughts occur, in the three-dimensional space in which your body sensations float? Can you imagine centering your awareness on the physical location of the source of thought in this three-dimensional body-space?

Can you imagine where in silence do the internal voices arise from? Where the visual images are located? Is it possible for you to imagine centering your awareness on the free flow of your thoughts and at the same time experience the physical space from which your thoughts issue, attending equally and simultaneously to the thoughts and to the spatial location from which thoughts emerge?

Can you imagine that as you center your awareness on the thoughts and the thinking process, and the location of the source of these thoughts, and the space in which this location exists, as you attend equally and simultaneously to the thoughts and their located source, can you imagine attending to the sense of self, self-awareness, as background?

Can you imagine this background awareness of self merging with the thoughts and the source of thought, simultaneously and equally imagining that this union is already in progress and is reaching its fulfillment, merging equally and simultaneously with source and thought and the space in which they occur?

And can you imagine that each time you become freshly aware of thought and the source of thought, you immediately merge your sense of self more evenly and more fully with thought and the source of the thought and the space in which they occur?

Can you imagine practicing this exercise during the day, while engaging in other activities or between activities?

Exercise

Seeing in Open Focus

INTRODUCTION

VISION IS the dominant sense in humans. Changing the way we attend to seeing the world is the most efficient way to diffuse stress. We can most quickly and effectively impact visual tensions and stresses by diffusing the scope of our vision and merging with all visual objects and space simultaneously aided by training.

This visual exercise guides us to change what we consider figure and what we consider ground, which can give us a clear experience of what moving in and out of narrow-objective focus and the associated tension changes feel like. Remember to give yourself fifteen seconds between questions to allow the described shifts of attention, of figure and ground, to happen.

PREPARATION

With eyes open, please sit in a gently erect posture while viewing a painting hanging at eye level. Alternatively, you can view a scene through a window. Any painting or window will do. A painting with a central figure would suffice.

GUIDING QUESTIONS

Can you imagine centering your attention on a chosen figure in the middle of the painting or window scene, something that stands out, and allowing into peripheral awareness the surround of the figure—that is, allowing all that is remaining on the painting or all of the remaining visible part of the scene, except for the chosen figure on which you're centered, to become the background of your visual awareness?

Can you imagine that throughout this exercise your eyes will be centered on this figure and that when other visual experience is mentioned you will diffuse the focus of your visual attention to include that material without redirecting the center of your visual awareness away from the figure?

Is it possible for you now to reverse this process of figure-and-ground awareness so that you allow the figure to recede and allow the background to move forward in your awareness, as if increasing your interest and the brightness of the background and reducing the interest in the figure as you allow it to recede? What was figure is now background. Without moving the direction of your gaze from the center of your view, what was background is now figure.

Is it possible for you now to attend equally to figure and ground so that the whole painting or scene is viewed equally and simultaneously, with no part of the painting or scene serving as figure or background for any other part?

Can you imagine now letting the whole painting or scene serve as figure and letting the wall on which the painting hangs or the wall on which the window is mounted serve as background?

Can you imagine now reversing this process and allowing the background wall to be highlighted in your awareness and letting the painting or the scene that was figure to recede, letting the painting or scene now serve as a background for seeing the surrounding wall as figure, again, without moving your eyes?

Is it possible for you now to attend equally to the painting or scene and the wall that contains or displays the window or painting so that neither serves as figure or ground for the other?

Is it possible for you to imagine now that the whole wall, including the painting or window, is figure and the side walls and the ceiling and the floor and all the people and objects in view are the background for seeing this front wall, including the painting or scene through the window, as the figure of your visual awareness?

Can you imagine now reversing this process, allowing all the objects in view—the side walls, the ceiling, and the floor—to serve as figure and allowing the front wall to be seen as the background for that experience, highlighting peripheral awareness as figure and central awareness as ground, again, without moving your eyes?

Can you imagine now attending to both the front wall and the surround—all the objects in view—equally and simultaneously so that no part of your visual experience serves as figure or ground for any other?

Can you imagine now attending to all of your experience of visual objects—people, furniture, other objects, the walls, the ceiling, the floor—as figure and allowing the space in which these objects exist and between and through these objects to serve as the background?

Can you imagine now reversing this process, attending to space as figure—you're more interested in the space than you are in the objects that exist in this space—and allowing the objects to be the background for your experience of space as figure?

Exercise

Can you imagine now attending equally and simultaneously to space and to everything that you can see?

Can you imagine now attending to the space and objects in your visual awareness as figure and allowing the sounds that occur in a three-dimensional space to serve as the background for seeing space and objects as figure?

Can you imagine now reversing this process, centering your attention on hearing silence and the sounds that occur in this silence and allowing visual experience of space and objects to serve as the background, the ground of experience?

Can you imagine now attending equally and simultaneously to seeing and hearing and the space and silence in which they occur so that neither serves as figure or ground for the other?

Can you imagine, again, now allowing the visual experience of space permeating the objects that occur in that space to serve as figure and allowing the feeling of presence of your whole body and any feelings or emotions that might be present and the feeling of space around and through your body and letting this feeling experience serve as background for seeing space and objects?

Can you imagine now reversing this process, letting the feeling experience of space and body and emotions serve as figure and letting visual experience of space and objects form the background for this experience of feeling?

160

Is it possible for you now to attend equally and simultaneously to seeing and feeling so that neither seeing nor feeling serves as figure or ground for the other?

Is it possible for you now to include also hearing silence and sounds so that seeing, hearing, and feeling are experienced simultaneously and equally?

Can you imagine now centering your attention on tasting and the space in which tastes occur and letting them serve as figure, and allowing seeing space and objects to serve as background for tasting?

Can you imagine now reversing this process, letting objects and space in visual awareness serve as figure and letting tastes and the space in which they occur serve as background for seeing?

Can you imagine now attending equally and simultaneously to visual and taste sensations and the space in which they occur?

Can you imagine now also including the sensations of feeling and hearing so that all four sensations—seeing, tasting, hearing, and feeling—and the common space-silence in which they occur are attended to equally and simultaneously?

Can you imagine now centering your attention on olfactory experience—smells, fragrances, odors, and the space in which they occur—as figure and letting seeing space and objects serve as the background for smelling?

Can you imagine now reversing this process so that seeing space and objects is figure and smelling space and odors is background?

Can you imagine experiencing seeing and smelling space and objects of sensation simultaneously and equally, neither serving as figure or ground for the other?

Can you imagine now including also tasting, feeling, and hearing so that all five ordinary senses are attended to simultaneously and equally, both the space common to them and their respective objects of sensation?

Can you imagine one homogeneous field of space in which these five senses simultaneously occur?

Can you imagine now attending to thinking—including visual imagery and internal dialogue and the space or void in which they occur—as figure and allowing seeing space and objects to serve as background?

Can you imagine now reversing this process and letting visual experience of space and objects serve as figure and allowing thinking and the space in which visual images occur or the silence in which internal dialogue occurs to serve as background?

Can you imagine now attending equally and simultaneously to visual objects and space and to thought objects and space?

Can you imagine now also including sensations of smell and taste and feeling and hearing so that all of these sense experiences and the space in which they occur represent one homogeneous field of experience, with none receiving more attention than the others?

Can you imagine basking or bathing in this simultaneous equal awareness of all senses and the space in which they occur, resting in this awareness?

Can you imagine now attending to sensations of presence—centered in nowness, experiencing oneself in this moment—bathed in the sensations of timelessness as figure and letting visual experience of space and objects serve as background?

Can you imagine reversing this process and using visual experience of object and space as figure and letting the sense of time and timelessness serve as background for seeing?

Can you imagine now attending equally to visual experience and temporal experience and space and timelessness equally and simultaneously?

Can you imagine now including also your other senses—the senses of smell and taste and hearing and feeling and the sense of mind or thought—and the space and silence in which they occur so that all seven of these senses represent one homogeneous and equally attended field of experience without figure or ground?

Can you imagine now attending to all of this—sensations and space in all seven sense modalities—as figure and allowing the sense organs, which give rise to their associated experiences, to serve as background so eyes and ears and body and tongue and nose and brain are experienced as the background for these homogeneously experienced sensations?

Can you imagine now reversing this process so that your sense experience and the space in which it occurs serve as the background for experiencing the sense organs and the space in which they occur as figure?

Can you imagine attending equally and simultaneously now to sensations and to the sense organs and to the space in which they occur?

Can you imagine attending to a sense of self, or self-awareness—the self that is aware of all of this—to serve as background for the multisensory experience of senses and sense organs and the space in which they occur as figure?

Can you imagine letting your sense of self or self-awareness serve as figure and letting all of your other experience—sensations and sense organs and the space in which they occur—serve as background for the sense of self?

Can you imagine letting this sense of self and the space in which it occurs and sensations and the organs of sensation and the space in which they occur all be attended to equally and simultaneously?

Can you imagine that this sense of self-awareness is already merging with the senses and their associated sense organs simultaneously and equally and also with the space in which they occur?

Can you imagine that when self-awareness is newly emerged into this moment that all your senses serve as background?

And can you imagine repeating this process until this recorded exercise ends or until this awareness, which is you, feels balanced and centered and is effortlessly merging with and emerging from all other experience present in the center and periphery of your awareness?

Can you imagine practicing this exercise or parts of this exercise repeatedly throughout each day?

Conclusion

THOUGHTS ON THE
EVOLUTION OF ATTENTION

*Man masters nature not by force
but by understanding.*

— JACOB BRONOWSKI,
Science and Human Values

AN AMOEBA floats in a sea of stimuli—light, temperature, vibration, touch, and chemicals. With primitive sense organs distributed over its membrane surface, even the lowly amoeba, with its ability to move toward some types of stimuli and away from others, shows some of the capacities of attention. An amoeba responds differently to a particle of food, for example, than to a speck of dust or a hot light.

All organisms, from the simplest to the most complex, are bombarded by stimulation. Single-celled organisms like the amoeba can only discriminate and respond in the most rudimentary ways to stimuli. However, as we move up the evolutionary tree, organisms exhibit higher and higher levels of organization, from the nerve nets of jellyfish to the nerve cords and ganglia of earthworms to the complex central and peripheral nervous systems of vertebrates, including humans. With this increased complexity of overarching anatomical structures dedicated to controlling lower level systems comes the evolution of the ability to attend in more subtle ways. This evolutionary drive to become more conscious, more aware of attention styles, makes possible conscious choice of attention styles, which can enhance and optimize performance.

It might reasonably be inferred that one of the major directions of evolution is toward improved mechanisms of attention. More and better information about its environment allows an organism to assess and select appropriate responses with greater precision. This process seems to have reached its apex in humans, who presumably have the most highly refined ability to discriminate among the world's creatures: Whereas an amoeba will engulf any food particles within a certain size range, humans prefer fruit of a certain appearance and of a distinct state of ripeness.

What truly sets us apart from all other forms of life, though—much more than our capacity for fine discrimination and subtle behavior—is the human ability to pay attention to how we attend. This ability stands at the apex of human evolution.

Attention skills allow us to alter our reality. We are, each of us, the creators of our lives in a very real sense. We can create a far different reality than the one we normally inhabit. We can build a world where we're more accepting and intimate and more loving, or more exclusive and distant.

One minute we can be an inclusive, loving being in Open Focus and the next an accountant paying attention exclusively to columns of numbers in narrow focus, an adversarial lawyer involved in conflict resolution, or an engineer working with detailed drawings. We can choose initially to objectify an experience and distance ourselves from it but then later decide to merge with it and experience it fully in a different way. And, of course, we can learn simultaneously to do both.

When we develop our attention skills, we can lay down our troubles and responsibilities at any time and leave them; or, if we want, we can take them up again. If we have anxiety, depression, or chronic physical pain, we can allow it to diffuse by changing the way we attend to it. Ultimately, by learning to use a variety of attention styles, we can free ourselves from the burden of the past and stop fretting about the future. We don't have to depend on others for our happiness or well-being. Nor are we subject to the tyranny of our unpleasant thoughts and feelings. We can discover a sense of freedom unlike any other.

Ripples in the Pond of the Brain

In my research into attention and EEG activity, one consistent pattern I've noticed has particularly interested me. As people rest in the present moment, central areas of the brain become synchronous, or in phase. However, the occipital (visual) region, remains persistently out of phase with other regions. I've seen this repeatedly in person after person. Over time, I've developed a theory about this observation that could help us to understand something about how the brain creates and dissolves our personal reality, how mental phenomena appear and disappear.[1]

Throw a stone into a pond and ripples in the water move outward. Throw two stones into a pond and waves will spread out from where each pebble was dropped. Where waves from the two dropped pebbles collide, a secondary pattern of moving waves is formed, something physicists call an interference pattern.

169

Conclusion

Consciousness might be said to consist of three primary elements: (1) attention, (2) the contents of our attention, and (3) the witness of both. Each of these elements is represented in the brain's electrical rhythms. The contents of attention are represented by activity in one or more sensory (for example, visual) regions of the brain, and attention (awareness) is represented by activity in much of the rest of the brain. When the activity between these regions is out of phase, then a distinction is made between internal and external attention content. When the activity is in phase between the two regions, then this distinction is lost, and these two elements are undifferentiated, becoming a unified whole. Out-of-phase activity between the two regions also creates an interference pattern where they abut, which is the mechanism that gives rise to the witnessing "self," the "I-am" self. Out-of-phase activity between regions allows us to separate self from attention and its contents, that is, from our surroundings. Animals and humans do this reflexively, but only humans can do it consciously. In narrow-objective focus the sense of self is most pronounced.

When we move into a more diffuse-immersed attention style, the self merges into attention and its contents, leading to more synchronous activity and increasing our ability to become volitionally unself-conscious. When attention and its contents brain activities are in phase, however, conscious distinctions disappear, because abutting brain regions do not create interference patterns. There is a lack of differentiation or separation between attention and its contents. All is one, and the self disappears.

Unself-consciousness is what happens, for example, when we arrive at our destination and can't remember driving ourselves there, or when we eat or do the dishes while our minds were not present. Certain tasks are so routine that we can perform them without staying aware of our awareness.

170

After learning how to access this state in Open-Focus training, one of my clients reported that previously she had only experienced it at the beach, her favorite place in the world. The great expanse of wide, sandy shore, the depth of vision to the horizon where ocean meets the vast blue sky, the smell of the sea, the breezes that rhythmically modulate the warmth of the sun as they caress the windward face of the skin—taken in simultaneously, all this would precipitate for her an experience of unself-consciousness and union. "I feel so small, even invisible, in this large space," she said.

The three-dimensional environments of beaches, mountains, oceans, deserts, and—for astronauts—space itself may evoke in us such changes in perception. Likewise, cathedrals, temples, museums, and other man-made structures can have the same effect. However, these geographical and architectural stimuli—as well as peak performance in artistic and athletic endeavors—are the occasion for, not the cause of, such experiences. With Open-Focus training, we learn that access to moments like these is not dependent on the presence of special conditions. Once we learn to shift into Open Focus, any situation can be the occasion for attentional release into unself-consciousness.[2]

At its most profound level, this lack of differentiation between self, attention and its contents, expands to a universal embrace, resulting in ecstatic experience, a sense of complete oneness.

The great physicist Werner Heisenberg said, "What we observe is not nature itself, but nature exposed to our method of questioning." Substitute the words "style of attention" for "method of questioning," and you have a statement that encapsulates the whole spirit of Open-Focus training. The way in which we frame our questions intimately depends on how we pay attention, and vice versa. It is my hope that learning about

171

Open Focus will allow readers to ask new questions, which will result in new answers.

Imagine the difference such a change could make in medical research and practice. As with narrow focus, the problem with medicine as currently practiced is not that it is precise, accurate, and objective but that it is only precise, accurate, and objective. "What is wrong with the brain?" "What is wrong with the body?" "How can we fix this machine and get it back on the road?" Driven by research funds from pharmaceutical companies and a cynical view of human health, these symptom-driven approaches have for too long been the questions dominating medical inquiry. The answer has been to expand the umbrella of pathology and make more medications.

The problem with an overdependence on medications is that they are a way of forcing the body to obey. The body and mind comprise a complex collection of systems. When we force changes on a small part of a system, when we don't understand it, there are unintended consequences, some of which may be apparent and some of which may not, at least not for many years. Time and again medicine has caused problems because we do not understand the many interactions between systems. Understanding attention offers us a new way of understanding the body's systems, rather than manipulating its components.

The human central nervous system is not broken in those instances—such as depression, anxiety, addictions, and ADHD, among others—where it is simply under stress. We must back away from reductionism and seek to promote organism-wide balance by quieting sympathetic autonomic activity, increasing parasympathetic activity, and asking what is *right* with the human body, mind, and spirit. The overuse of narrow-objective attention got us into our current epidemic of stress-related problems, and relearning how to rebalance attention processes can get us out. We need to master brain function and its connection to other aspects of human physiology, to paraphrase Bronowski, less by forcing it to bend to our will and more through opening to our experience and understanding.

INDEPENDENCE DAY

Open Focus is available to everyone, to deepen their life experiences, no matter what those experiences might be. It isn't meant to compete with other techniques of self-management. It doesn't conflict with any philosophy, religion, science, culture, or personal value system.

People going through life with the flexible awareness of Open Focus—perhaps with daily attention training at work, school, or home—will open their hearts to the fullness of their being, and reintegrate forgotten parts of themselves. The brain is built to learn throughout our life span; current research on neural plasticity is proving that. With enough training and practice, learning to flexibly shift attention becomes effortless and natural. Flexible attention permits us to move in and out of full rest, allowing our body to restore itself and thus prevent and heal many stress-based problems common today. Think back to the pride of lions in chapter 2—how effortless their repose was after the fierce concentration of the hunt. We have that same ability; and once we have reclaimed it, we can so much better use those faculties that are uniquely human.

What would happen if an Olympic swimmer were wrapped in a full-body bandage and dropped in a turbulent river? She wouldn't stand a chance. Just as the bandage would prevent the swimmer from using her superior abilities in the water, so does our being locked in narrow-objective focus constrain us from using our natural range of attention styles to successfully navigate and use to our best advantage the overwhelming torrent of stimuli that confronts us each day. So rather than taking an active role in creating our lives, we are reduced to coping with them. This is not how things could be. We are able to live creatively, spontaneously, and flexibly. The day we learn to do so is our true Independence Day.

Can you imagine a world where we are all living in Open Focus, dissolving our pain, anxiety, restlessness, boredom, uncertainty, and chronic dissatisfaction? Can you imagine a world where we are free from the tyranny of mental content, dwelling in the spacious context of our awareness? Can you imagine freely giving and receiving love, merging with the world instead of feeling isolated and separate from it, and sensing and experiencing the world also as the wondrous place that it is? This is possible only when we assume fully our role as attender and practice a flexible deployment of attention.

Epilogue

The biggest deterrent to scientific progress is a refusal
of some people, including scientists, to believe that
things that seem amazing can really happen.

— GEORGE TRIMBLE, Director, NASA
Manned Spacecraft Center

As you finish this book, it might seem that Open Focus is too good to be true, too easy. Rest assured. While we have written about some of the cases with the most satisfactory resolution here, everything written is true to the best of our knowledge. Each anecdote is from a real person (though names were changed for privacy's sake) and the results are the kind we see frequently.

When, by happenstance, I meet past clients or previous students of Open Focus, they almost invariably praise their involvement with Open-Focus attention training. The benefits are clear to them. When I ask how often they still engage in home practice they say "not enough." When I persist, they confess that they practice hardly at all, unless a new problem arises, causing them to narrow focus and overreact, pushing them to respond with old rigid habits of attention. To restore balance they say they practice until they regain attention flexibility, then practice trails off. This, for the most part, is how many longtime users of Open Focus use it—like a pill they take when they feel stress symptoms.

Open Focus is a centered way of being, but the people whose cases are written in this book—and many, many, others—are the ones who put in the time and did their homework. My own fervent wish is that students of Open Focus develop a desire to take Open Focus all the way, as a life journey, as a daily art, gradually deepening styles of attention and increasing flexibility of application.

Notes

CHAPTER 1: An Addiction to Narrow Focus

1. H. G. Hoffman, J. N. Doctor, D. R. Patterson, G. J. Carrougher, and T.A. Furness, III, "Use of Virtual Reality for Adjunctive Treatment of Adolescent Burn Pain During Wound Care: A Case Report," *Pain* 85 (2000): 305–9.

CHAPTER 2: Sweet Surrender: Discovering the Benefits of Synchronous Alpha Brain Waves

1. Lester G. Fehmi, J. W. Adkins, and Donald B. Lindsley, "Electrophysiological Correlates of Visual Perceptual Masking in Monkeys," *Experimental Brain Research* 7 (1969): 299–316.

2. See L. Gannon and R. Sternbach, "Alpha Enhancement as a Treatment for Pain: A Case Study, *Behavior Therapy and Experimental Psychiatry* 2 (1971): 209–13; K. Pelletier and E. Peper, "Developing a Biofeedback Model: Alpha EEG Feedback as a Means for Pain Control, *International Journal of Clinical and Experimental Hypnosis* 25, no. 4 (1977): 361–71; E. G. Peniston and P. J. Kulkosky, "Alpha Theta Brainwave Training for Vietnam Veterans with Combat-Related Post Traumatic Stress Disorder," *Medical Psychotherapy* 4 (1991): 47–60; Peniston and Kulkosky, "Alcoholic Personality and Alpha Theta Brain Wave Training," *Medical Psychotherapy* 3 (1990): 37–55; J. T. McKnight and Les Fehmi, "Attention and Neurofeedback Synchrony Training: Clinical Results and Their Significance," *Journal of Neurotherapy* 5, nos. 1–21 (2001): 45–62; D. Lehmann, W. Lang, and P. Debruyne, "Controlled EEG Alpha Feedback Training in Normals and Headache Patients," *Archives of Psychiatry* 221 (1976): 331–43; A. Matthew, H. Mishm, and

V. Kumamiah, "Alpha Feedback in the Treatment of Tension Headache," *Journal of Personality and Clinical Studies* 3, no. 1 (1987): 17–22; Hanslmayr, Sausing, Doppelmayr, Schabus, and Klimerer, "Increasing Individual Upper Alpha Power by Neurofeedback Improves Cognitive Performance in Human Subjects," *Applied Psychophysiology and Biofeedback* 30, no. 1 (2005).

3. See Ernst Niebur, Steven S. Hsiao, and Kenneth O. Johnson, "Synchrony: A Neuronal Mechanism for Attentional Selection?" *Current Opinion in Neurobiology* 12, no. 2 (2002): 190–95. Also of interest is Pascal Fries, John H. Reynolds, Alan E. Rorie, and Robert Desimone, "Modulation of Oscillatory Neuronal Synchronization by Selective Visual Attention," *Science* 291, no. 5508 (2001): 1560–63. Desimone, Fries, and their colleagues believe that synchronous neuronal firing may be a fundamental mechanism for boosting the volume of brain signals representing behaviorally relevant stimuli and that many mental disorders are due to the brain's inability to fire synchronously.

4. William Tiller, *Science and Human Transformation: Subtle Energies, Intentionality and Consciousness* (Walnut Creek, Calif.: Pavior Publishing, 1997). Also, "The tendency to synchronize," writes Steven Strogatz, a professor of applied mathematics at Cornell University, in his book *Sync: How Order Emerges from Chaos in the Universe, Nature and Daily Life*, "may be the most mysterious and pervasive drive in all of nature."

5. Numerous EEG studies have shown increased synchrony in meditators. See Michael Murphy and Steven Donovan, *The Physical and Psychological Effects of Meditation: A Review of Contemporary Research with a Comprehensive Bibliography, 1931–1996*, 2nd ed. (Petaluma, CA: Institute of Noetic Sciences, 1997). According to that book's editors, "EEG synchronization/coherence with respect to the distribution of alpha activity between the four anatomically distinct regions of the brain—left, right, anterior and posterior—may indicate the effectiveness of meditation."

6. James V. Hardt and Joseph Kamiya, "Anxiety Change through EEG Alpha Feedback: Seen Only in High-Anxiety Subjects," *Science* 201 (1978): 79–81.

7. For research indicating that phase coherence is associated with clear or "pure" thinking, see K. Badawi, R. K. Wallace, A. M. Rouzere, and D. Orme-Johnson, "Electrophysical Changes during Periods of Respiratory Suspension in the Transcendental Meditation Technique," *Psychosomatic Medicine* 46 (1984): 267–76. An earlier study that arrived at similar findings is J. T. Farrow and J. R. Herbert, "Breath Suspension During the Transcendental Meditation Technique," *Psychosomatic Medicine* 44, no. 2 (1982): 133–53. These same studies also found that alpha synchrony increases in long-term meditators.

CHAPTER 3: The Full Complement of Attention

1. George Fritz and Les Fehmi, *The Open-Focus Handbook* (Princeton: Biofeedback Computers, 1982), 33.
2. Nearly thirty studies support this correlation, which was first recognized by Eugene Gendlin of the University of Chicago. For a review of these studies, see L. S. Greenberg and W. M. Pinsof, *The Psychotherapeutic Process: A Research Handbook* (New York: Guilford Press, 1986), 21–71.
3. George Fritz and Les Fehmi, *The Open-Focus Handbook* (Princeton: Biofeedback Computers, 1982), 15.
4. Ibid., 27.
5. Ibid.
6. Ibid., 28–29.

Exercise: A Feeling of Space

1. The "homunculus" is a miniature "person" represented in each half (hemisphere) of the brain. The feet start at the top in the middle of the head, and the parts of the body are inverted from there down to the sides. The size of the brain area devoted to each region is related to the sensitivity and degree of control we have over those parts.

CHAPTER 4: What Lies Beneath: Anxiety

1. See Lisa Kalynchuk et al., "Corticosterone Increases Depression-Like Behavior with Some Effects on Predator Odor-Induced

Defensive Behavior in Male and Female Rats," *Behavioral Neuro-science* 118 (2004): 1365–77.

2. Understanding the regions of the brain active in face and object recognition is a large area of research, and hundreds of studies have tried to parse the different brain regions involved. Researchers with the Kodak company discovered that when people with ADHD are made to look at a blank computer screen, their fingertip temperatures quickly drop. "The lack of stimulation increases and his or her level of anxiety and stress level increases." The discovery led Kodak to develop a diagnostic tool for ADHD that measures fingertip temperature.

3. Bruce D. Perry, "The Memories of States: How the Brain Stores and Retrieves Traumatic Experiences," in *Splintered Reflections: Images of the Body in Trauma,"* ed. Jean Goodwin and Reina Attias (New York: Basic Books, 1999).

4. Meredith F. Small, "Family Matters," *Discover* 21, no. 8 (2000).

5. Ibid.

6. William S. Condon and Louis W. Sander, "Neonate Movement Is Synchronized with Adult Speech: Interactional Participation and Language Acquisition," *Science* 183, no. 4120 (1974): 99–101.

CHAPTER 5: Dissolving Physical Pain

1. See H. G. Fassbender and K. Wegner, "Morphologie und Pathogenese des Weichteilrheumatismus," *Z. Rheumaforsch* 32 (1973): 355, cited in John Sarno, *Mind Over Back Pain* (New York: Berkeley Books, 1982). In his book, Dr. Sarno, a New York University physician, gives an excellent account of how severe muscle pain is caused by the repressed contents of the unconscious.

CHAPTER 6: Dissolving Emotional Pain

1. John Furness, *The Enteric Nervous System* (Malden, Mass.: Blackwell, 2005).

2. No one knows precisely how attention to our visual experience affects us so deeply and so globally, but there is some research to suggest a possible mechanism. In the 1980s two researchers at Harvard Medical School, Dr. Margaret Livingstone and Dr. David Hubel (whose work on information processing in the visual system

earned him and a colleague the Nobel Prize for Medicine in 1981) discovered that the visual system connects to the brain via two distinct, parallel pathways, called the parvocellular and magnocellular. Parvo cells are found exclusively at the center of the visual field, while the peripheral visual field contains a mix of both magno and parvo cells. These two systems are present throughout the visual apparatus, from the retina to the cortex.

Some believe that these two channels have very different functions in the central nervous system. Joseph Trachtman, PhD, a Brooklyn psychologist and optometrist who treats ADHD and visual problems by retraining vision, believes the parvo cells in the center of the retina activate high-frequency beta brain waves, and the magno cells in the outer ring of the retina engage amplified alpha and theta brain waves. In other words, attending with the central part of the eye engages mostly high-frequency EEG activity, while emphasizing attention to the peripheral fields of experience—as in diffuse attention—engages the magno cells and a lower range of frequencies. Trachtman also believes that parvo cells are linked directly to the left brain and therefore with logical and analytical thinking and sustained visual tasks. He believes the magno cells are wired to the right hemisphere, which governs creativity, three-dimensional perception, and visceral feelings. Using biofeedback, Trachtman treats myopia and ADHD by teaching clients to engage the outer part of the retina. He reports that the treatment also results in marked positive changes in emotions, improved immune system function, and reduced muscle tension. The implication seems to be that in order for the cognitive and emotional aspects of the brain to function appropriately, both the inner and outer parts of the eye and both hemispheres of the brain need to be used simultaneously.

There has long been a small but committed school of thought that holds that learning and behavioral problems are exacerbated by vision problems, an idea advanced by Dr. A. M. Skeffington, father of behavioral optometry and cofounder of the Optometric Extension Program in Santa Ana, California. Before Hubel and Livingstone confirmed it, Skeffington had claimed that there are two parts to the visual pathway and that learning to use both central and peripheral visual subsystems was an effective way of teaching children to calm themselves and to overcome ADHD and other learning problems. He found that teaching children to change the way they attend to visual experience did more than change their vision—it also helped to resolve a range of emotional and cognitive problems.

A number of other behavioral approaches, including the venerable Bates method, hold that many eye problems have their origin in emotional and physical stress. Chronic tension in the eye muscles pulls the eye out of its natural shape, a distortion that impairs vision. Adherents of these methods use a number of attention-changing exercises (though they don't call them that) to help the eye regain its original shape and function.

In San Bernadino, California, Stanley Kaseno, a developmental optometrist, has successfully treated juvenile delinquents solely with optometry. In one study researchers examined one thousand delinquents and found that only 5 percent had normal visual perceptual systems. They prescribed 451 pairs of glasses to subjects who needed them but had never had them prescribed. They prescribed therapy that included a number of vision-related exercises, including visual imagery, visual memory, and locating objects in space. At the end of the study, using only visual therapies, the average sixteen-year-old had raised his level of reading from grade 5 to grade 8.5 and his measured IQ from ninety to ninety-five. Moreover the rate of rearrest of these teenagers dropped from between 50 and 60 percent to 10 percent.

3. There are volumes of studies on the effects of emotional stress on the immune system. See Bruce S. Rabin, *Stress, Immune Function, and Health: The Connection* (New York: Wiley, 1999).

CHAPTER 7: Love Is a Way of Paying Attention: Open-Focus Tools for Relationships
Exercise: Heart-Centered Open Focus
1. The HeartMath Institute has done a great deal of research on the role of the heart in human psychology. See Rollin McCraty, Mike Atkinson, and Dana Tomasino, *Science of the Heart: Exploring the Role of the Heart in Human Performance: An Overview of Research*

Conducted by the Institute of HeartMath (Boulder Creek, Calif.: Institute of HeartMath, 2001), www.heartmath.org/research/ science-of-the-heart/index.html.

2. There is a great deal of research on heart disease and depression. A Montreal Heart Institute study with 222 subjects found that depressed heart-attack survivors are four times more likely to die within six months than their nondepressed counterparts. See N. Frasure-Smith, F. Lesperance, and M. Talajic, "Depression Following Myocardial Infarction: Impact on Six-Month Survival," *Journal of the American Medical Association* 270, no. 15 (1993): 1819–25.

   A Johns Hopkins study involving 1,551 people concluded that depressed people are four times more likely to have a heart attack. See Laura A. Pratt et al., "Depression, Psychotropic Medication, and Risk of Myocardial Infarction: Prospective Data from the Baltimore ECA Follow-Up," *Circulation* 94 (1996): 3123–29.

   At Ohio State University researchers found that depressed men were 70 percent more likely to develop heart disease. See Amy K. Ferketich et al., "Depression as an Antecedent to Heart Disease among Women and Men in the NHANES I Study," *Archives of Internal Medicine* 160 (2000): 1261–68.

CHAPTER 8: Peak Performance

1. Dan Landers et al., "Hemispheric Asymmetry, Cardiac Response, and Performance in Elite Archers," *Research Quarterly for Exercise and Sport* 61, no. 4 (1990): 351–59.
2. See M. Kavussanu, D. J. Crews, and D. L. Gill, "The Effects of Single versus Multiple Measures of Biofeedback on Basketball Free Throw Shooting Performance," *International Journal of Sport Psychology* 29, no. 2 (1998): 132–44. See also Gavin M. Loze, David Collins, and Paul S. Holmes, "Pre-Shot EEG Alpha-Power Reactivity during Expert Air-Pistol Shooting: A Comparison of Best and Worst Shots," *Journal of Sports Sciences* 19, no. 9 (2001): 727–33.
3. Dan Landers et al., "The Influence of Electrocortical Biofeedback in Performance in Pre-Elite Archers," *Medicine and Science in Sports and Exercise* 23 (1991): 123–29.
4. Tobias Egner and John H. Gruzelier, "Ecological Validity of

Neurofeedback: Modulation of Slow-Wave EEG Enhances Musical Performance," *Neuroreport* 14, no. 9 (2003): 1221–24.

CHAPTER 9: Living in Open Focus
1. Turk, et al., "The Distributed Nature of the Self," *Annals of the New York Academy of Sciences* 1001 (Oct. 2003).
2. George Fritz and Les Fehmi, *The Open-Focus Handbook* (Princeton: Biofeedback Computers, 1982), 101.

CHAPTER 10: Attention and Psychotherapy
1. In fact, this shift now seems to be under way in the practice of psychotherapy, as evidenced by the popularity of and growing research base for Acceptance and Commitment Therapy, Dialectical Behavior Therapy, and Mindfulness-Based Cognitive Therapy, all of which emphasize working with the process and overall context of awareness rather than simply trying to understand and modify or control mental content.

CONCLUSION: Thoughts on Attention and Reality
1. A more detailed account of this theory is presented at www.Open Focus.com.
2. George Fritz and Les Fehmi, *The Open-Focus Handbook* (Princeton: Biofeedback Computers, 1982), 132–33.

Index

Index

About the Authors

A PIONEER in the field of neurofeedback, LES FEHMI, PHD, BCIA-EEG, is director of the Princeton Biofeedback Center in Princeton, New Jersey. He holds an MA and PhD in psychology from UCLA and completed his post-doctoral fellowship at UCLA's Brain Research Institute. An affiliate member of the Department of Medicine at Princeton University Medical Center, over the past four decades Dr. Fehmi has been active as a psychologist in private practice, a speaker, and an author in peer-reviewed journals. A certified "speed-and-explosion specialist," Dr. Fehmi has worked with the Dallas Cowboys, the New Jersey Nets, and the Olympic Development Committee. He has also served as a consultant for Harvard's Massachusetts General Hospital, the Johnson & Johnson corporation, and the Veterans Administration. This is his first book for a general audience.

For more information on Dr. Les Fehmi and Open-Focus training, or to order a complete set of Open-Focus exercises on audio CD, visit www.openfocus.com. Research articles are also available there for download.

JIM ROBBINS is an award-winning journalist and science writer, with frequent contributions to the *New York Times, Smithsonian, Scientific American, Discover,* and *Psychology*

Today. In connection with his reporting, he has appeared on ABC's *Nightline* and NPR's *All Things Considered* and *Morning Edition*. He is also the author of *A Symphony in the Brain: The Evolution of the New Brain Wave Biofeedback*, which was excerpted in *Newsweek* and the *New York Times*.